The Fertility Solution

The Fertility Solution

Fertility Secrets for the Modern Woman Over 40

By

Zahra C. Franklin

Disclaimer

"The Fertility Solution: Fertility Secrets for the Modern Woman Over 40" contains advice and material that is solely meant for general educational purposes. Zahra Franklin, the author, does not hold a license as a psychologist, therapist, or medical practitioner. It is recommended that readers seek the counsel of certified experts for individualized guidance and assistance catered to their specific situations.

Any liability resulting from the use of this guide, whether direct or indirect, is disclaimed by the author and publisher. The author and publisher have taken every care to assure the authenticity of the information; however, they cannot guarantee that the content is adequate or complete. The reader assumes full responsibility for their actions based on the information provided in this guide.

About the Author

Zahra C. Franklin is a renowned fertility specialist, author, and advocate for women's reproductive health and empowerment. With over two decades of experience in the field of fertility medicine, Zahra has dedicated her career to helping women overcome challenges and achieve their dreams of motherhood, particularly those navigating the journey after the age of 40.

In addition to her clinical work, Zahra is deeply committed to education and outreach. She regularly speaks at seminars and workshops, sharing her expertise and empowering women with the knowledge they need to make informed decisions about their fertility journey. Zahra's compassionate approach and dedication to patient care have earned her the trust and gratitude of countless individuals and families worldwide.

"The Fertility Solution: Fertility Secrets for the Modern Woman Over 40" is Zahra's latest endeavor to provide women with practical guidance, evidence-based strategies, and inspirational stories to navigate the complexities of fertility in today's world. Through her writing, Zahra aims to demystify the process of fertility treatment, offer hope and encouragement, and empower women to take control of their reproductive health.

Table of Contents

INTRODUCTION

In recent years, there has been a notable shift in the landscape of family planning, with more and more women choosing to embark on the journey of motherhood later in life. This trend reflects a myriad of societal, cultural, and personal factors that influence the decision-making process surrounding family formation. Whether it's pursuing career aspirations, prioritizing personal growth, or simply waiting for the right partner, the reasons behind this shift are as diverse as the women themselves.

Gone are the days when women were expected to marry young and start a family shortly thereafter. Today, women are embracing the freedom to chart their own paths and make informed choices about their reproductive timelines. With advancements in healthcare, education, and career opportunities, many women are delaying pregnancy until their 30s and even 40s, redefining the traditional notions of motherhood and fertility.

This phenomenon is not limited to any one demographic or geographic region but is rather a global trend observed across various cultures and socioeconomic backgrounds. From urban professionals to suburban mothers, women from all walks of life are reevaluating the timeline for starting a family and embracing the concept of "delayed motherhood" as a viable option.

However, despite the growing acceptance of delayed motherhood, there remain prevalent misconceptions and challenges surrounding fertility after 40. One of the most pervasive myths is the belief that a woman's fertility drops off sharply once she reaches her 40s, making conception nearly impossible. While it's true that fertility declines with age, the reality is far more nuanced, with many women successfully conceiving and carrying healthy pregnancies well into their 40s and beyond.

Moreover, societal pressures and stigmas often exacerbate the emotional burden faced by women navigating fertility in their 40s. The fear of judgment, the pressure to conceive quickly, and the relentless barrage of well-meaning but often unsolicited advice can take a toll on one's mental and emotional well-being, introducing even another level of difficulty to a journey that is already difficult.

In this book, we will embark on a journey of discovery and empowerment, debunking myths, dispelling misconceptions, and equipping women with the knowledge, tools, and strategies they need to maximize their fertility potential after 40. Drawing on the latest research, expert insights, and real-life experiences, we will explore a holistic approach to fertility enhancement that encompasses nutrition, lifestyle optimization, cutting-edge technologies, and holistic therapies.

From practical tips for optimizing fertility to coping strategies for navigating emotional challenges, each chapter will be a beacon of hope and empowerment for women on their fertility journey. Through inspiring stories of triumph and resilience, readers will find solace, encouragement, and the unwavering belief that motherhood after 40 is not only possible but also within reach.

As we embark on this transformative journey together, let us embrace the power of knowledge, resilience, and unwavering hope, knowing that the path to motherhood knows no age limits and that every woman has the potential to unlock the fertility solution within her.

Throughout the pages of this book, we will delve deep into the complexities of fertility after 40, navigating the terrain with empathy, understanding, and unwavering support. We will confront the challenges head-on, armed with evidence-based information and practical advice tailored specifically for the modern woman over 40.

But beyond the statistics and medical jargon lies a profound truth: the journey to motherhood is as much a spiritual and emotional one as it is a physical one. It's about embracing the unknown, surrendering to the process, and trusting in the inherent wisdom of the body.

As we embark on this journey together, I invite you to approach each page with an open heart and a curious mind, ready to explore new possibilities, challenge old beliefs, and accept the limitless potential that you possess.

Together, we will uncover the fertility secrets that have eluded us for so long, unlocking the door to a future filled with hope, possibility, and the boundless joys of motherhood.

So let us begin this journey of discovery, empowerment, and transformation, knowing that no matter where it leads us, we are never alone. For in the sisterhood of women, united by a common dream, lies the greatest source of strength, support, and solidarity.

Welcome to "The Fertility Solution: Fertility Secrets for the Modern Woman Over 40." May it be a beacon of light, hope, and empowerment on your journey to motherhood.

CHAPTER 1

Understanding Fertility After 40

Navigating fertility after the age of 40 presents unique challenges and considerations for women embarking on the journey to motherhood. It's crucial to understand the biological changes that occur in the body as women age and how these changes can impact fertility.

First and foremost, it's important to recognize that fertility naturally declines with age. As women enter their 40s, they experience a decrease in the quantity and quality of their eggs, making conception more challenging. This decline in fertility is primarily attributed to age-related changes in the ovaries, including a decrease in ovarian reserve and an increase in chromosomal abnormalities in eggs.

However, while fertility may decline with age, it's not impossible for women in their 40s to conceive. With advancements in reproductive technologies and medical interventions, many women are able to overcome age-related fertility barriers and achieve successful pregnancies.

Additionally, it's essential to consider other factors that can impact fertility, such as overall health, lifestyle choices, and underlying medical conditions. Factors like smoking, excessive alcohol consumption, obesity, and certain medical conditions can further diminish fertility and increase the risk of pregnancy complications.

Understanding fertility after 40 involves not only acknowledging the biological realities but also empowering women with knowledge, support, and resources to maximize their fertility potential. By taking proactive steps to optimize health, address lifestyle factors, and explore fertility treatment options, women can navigate the challenges of fertility after 40 with confidence and resilience. Ultimately, with the right support and guidance, women in their 40s can embark on the journey to motherhood with hope and determination.

Explaining the Biological Changes in a Woman's Body After 40

As women age, their bodies undergo a series of biological changes that can significantly impact fertility and reproductive health. These changes are influenced by a complex interplay of hormonal shifts, genetic factors, and environmental influences. Understanding these biological changes is crucial for women navigating fertility after the age of 40, as it can inform decisions regarding family planning, fertility treatment options, and overall reproductive health management.

1. Ovarian Aging

One of the most significant biological changes that occur in a woman's body after the age of 40 is ovarian aging. The ovaries, which are responsible for producing eggs and regulating reproductive hormones, undergo a gradual decline in function as women approach menopause. This decline is characterized by a decrease in the number and quality of eggs, a process known as ovarian reserve decline.

As women age, the number of follicles, which contain immature eggs, decreases, leading to a reduction in ovarian reserve. Additionally, the quality of the remaining eggs may diminish, increasing the risk of chromosomal abnormalities and pregnancy complications. This decline in ovarian function can make it more difficult for women over 40 to conceive naturally and may necessitate fertility treatments such as in vitro fertilization (IVF) or egg donation.

2. Hormonal Changes

Alongside ovarian aging, women experience significant hormonal changes as they enter perimenopause and menopause. Perimenopause typically begins in the late 30s to early 40s and is characterized by irregular menstrual cycles, fluctuating hormone levels, and symptoms such as hot flashes, night sweats, and mood swings.

During perimenopause, levels of reproductive hormones such as estrogen and progesterone fluctuate unpredictably, leading to disruptions in the menstrual cycle and ovulation. These hormonal fluctuations can further contribute to fertility challenges and may impact the success of fertility treatments.

As women transition into menopause, typically around the age of 50, ovarian function ceases altogether, leading to the cessation of menstruation and the end of reproductive capacity. This hormonal shift marks the end of the fertile window and signifies the onset of a new phase of life for women.

3. Changes in Reproductive Anatomy

In addition to ovarian aging and hormonal changes, women may also experience changes in their reproductive anatomy as they age. These changes can include alterations in the structure and function of the uterus, cervix, and fallopian tubes, which may impact fertility and pregnancy outcomes.

For example, changes in cervical mucus production and quality can affect sperm motility and transport, making it more difficult for sperm to reach and fertilize an egg. Similarly, age-related changes in the uterine lining can impact implantation and the ability to sustain a pregnancy.

Additionally, the risk of gynecological conditions such as fibroids, endometriosis, and polycystic ovary syndrome (PCOS) may increase with age, further complicating fertility and reproductive health. These conditions can interfere with ovulation, fertilization, and embryo implantation, requiring medical intervention to address.

4. Genetic Factors

Another important consideration in understanding fertility after 40 is the role of genetic factors in reproductive aging. Genetic predispositions, inherited traits, and chromosomal abnormalities can influence a woman's fertility potential and reproductive health outcomes as she ages.

For example, certain genetic mutations or chromosomal abnormalities may increase the risk of early menopause or ovarian dysfunction, impacting fertility at a younger age. Conversely, genetic factors may also play a role in determining the rate of ovarian aging and the onset of menopause, influencing the timing of fertility decline in individual women.

Additionally, genetic testing and screening may be recommended for women considering fertility treatments or assisted reproductive technologies, as certain genetic conditions can impact the success rates and outcomes of these interventions.

5. Metabolism and Weight

Slower Metabolism because as we age, our body's ability to burn calories naturally decreases. This can contribute to weight gain, even if eating habits remain unchanged. And Body Composition change as fat distribution tends to shift after 40, with more fat accumulating around the abdomen and less in the hips and thighs.

6. Musculoskeletal System

As advance in age one's Bone Density Loss because Women experience a more rapid decline in bone density after menopause due to decreased estrogen levels, increasing the risk of osteoporosis and their Muscle mass naturally declines with age, leading to decreased strength and endurance.

7. Skin:

Women in their 40's Skin loses collagen and elastin, leading to wrinkles and sagging and Hair growth may slow down, and hair may become thinner or grayer.so also are their risk of heart disease increases after menopause due to hormonal changes and other factors.

8. Environmental and Lifestyle Factors

In addition to biological and genetic factors, environmental and lifestyle factors can also influence fertility and reproductive health outcomes in women over 40. Factors such as smoking, excessive alcohol consumption, obesity, and exposure to environmental toxins can all negatively impact ovarian function, hormone levels, and overall fertility.

Smoking, for example, has been shown to accelerate ovarian aging and decrease ovarian reserve, making it more difficult for women to conceive and increasing the risk of infertility. Similarly, obesity and poor dietary habits can disrupt hormonal balance, interfere with ovulation, and impair fertility.

Conversely, adopting a healthy lifestyle that includes regular exercise, a balanced diet, stress management, and avoidance of harmful substances can help support reproductive health and optimize fertility outcomes. Lifestyle modifications may also enhance the success of fertility treatments and improve pregnancy outcomes for women over 40.

In summary, understanding the biological changes that occur in a woman's body after the age of 40 is essential for women navigating fertility and reproductive health in their later reproductive years. From ovarian aging and hormonal shifts to changes in reproductive anatomy and genetic factors, a myriad of factors can influence fertility potential and pregnancy outcomes in women over 40.

By acknowledging and addressing these biological changes, women can make informed decisions about family planning, fertility treatment options, and lifestyle modifications to support reproductive health. Moreover, healthcare providers and fertility specialists can tailor interventions and support services to meet the unique needs of women in this age group, offering hope, guidance, and compassionate care on their fertility journey.

Ultimately, while fertility may decline with age, it's important for women to remember that every individual's fertility journey is unique, and there are often options and solutions available to help achieve their reproductive goals. With knowledge, support, and proactive management of reproductive health, women over 40 can embark on the journey to motherhood with confidence, resilience, and optimism for the future.

Debunking myths and misconceptions surrounding fertility in older women

Women are sometimes subjected to myths and misconceptions regarding fertility as they get older, especially when it comes to getting pregnant later in life. These false beliefs have the potential to cause needless worry, anxiety, and misunderstanding, which keeps women from making knowledgeable decisions regarding their reproductive health. In this part, we'll bust some of the most widespread misconceptions about older women's fertility and offer fact-based analysis to correct false information.

Myth 1: Natural conception is impossible for women over 40.

One of the most widespread misconceptions about older women's fertility is this one, and it's just untrue. Many women in their 40s are still able to conceive spontaneously and have healthy children, despite the fact that fertility does decrease with age. The natural pregnancy rate for women between the ages of 40 and 44 is roughly 7% per month, which may be less than for younger women but is still quite probable, according to study published in the journal Human Reproduction.

It's critical to understand that there are large individual variations in fertility, and that a woman's ability for conception can be influenced by a variety of factors, including her general health, her lifestyle, and her genetic makeup. Age is a major contributing factor to the loss in fertility, although it is not the only factor in determining successful reproduction.

Myth 2: Women over 40 can only conceive through IVF.

For women over 40 who are having trouble conceiving, in vitro fertilization (IVF) is one option, but it is not the only one accessible. A lot of women in their 40s can still become pregnant spontaneously, particularly if they are healthy and don't have any underlying reproductive problems. Furthermore, depending on each woman's unique situation, further fertility therapies including ovulation induction and intrauterine insemination (IUI) may be appropriate.

It is imperative that women seek advice from a fertility specialist in order to investigate all of their choices and create a customized treatment plan. Whether using assisted reproductive technologies or natural means, women can improve their chances of conceiving and having a healthy pregnancy by adopting a comprehensive approach to fertility treatment and treating any underlying issues that may be influencing reproductive health.

Myth 3: Women over 40 have a significantly increased chance of miscarrying.

Even though the chance of miscarriage does rise with age, particularly after 35, it's crucial to remember that most pregnancies in women over 40 still end happily. The American College of Obstetricians and Gynecologists (ACOG) reports that the chance of miscarriage is over 34% for women in their 40s and 44s, vs approximately 10-12% for women in their 20s and early 30s.Despite the frightening nature of these numbers, it's important to keep in mind that many women in their 40s go on to have successful pregnancies and children. Additionally, improvements in prenatal care and genetic screening can help detect and reduce any dangers, giving women the resources and support they need to succeed.

Navigating fertility after the age of 40 presents unique challenges and considerations for women embarking on the journey to motherhood. It's crucial to understand the biological changes that occur in the body as women age and how these changes can impact fertility.

First and foremost, it's important to recognize that fertility naturally declines with age. As women enter their 40s, they experience a decrease in the quantity and quality of their eggs, making conception more challenging. This decline in fertility is primarily attributed to age-related changes in the ovaries, including a decrease in ovarian reserve and an increase in chromosomal abnormalities in eggs.

However, while fertility may decline with age, it's not impossible for women in their 40s to conceive. With advancements in reproductive technologies and medical interventions, many women are able to overcome age-related fertility barriers and achieve successful pregnancies.

Additionally, it's essential to consider other factors that can impact fertility, such as overall health, lifestyle choices, and underlying medical conditions. Factors like smoking, excessive alcohol consumption, obesity, and certain medical conditions can further diminish fertility and increase the risk of pregnancy complications.

Understanding fertility after 40 involves not only acknowledging the biological realities but also empowering women with knowledge, support, and resources to maximize their fertility potential. By taking proactive steps to optimize health, address lifestyle factors, and explore fertility treatment options, women can navigate the challenges of fertility after 40 with confidence and resilience. Ultimately, with the right support and guidance, women in their 40s can embark on the journey to motherhood with hope and determination.

Myth 4: Children born to older mothers are more likely to have birth problems.

Although there is a correlation between maternal age and the likelihood of specific chromosomal disorders, such Down syndrome, the overall risk is still rather low. As opposed to 1 in 1,250 at age 25, the Centers for Disease Control and Prevention (CDC) estimates that the chance of having a child with Down syndrome at age 40 is about 1 in 100.

It's crucial to remember that the great majority of infants born to older moms are healthy and defect-free. Furthermore, chromosomal abnormalities can now be detected early in pregnancy thanks to advancements in prenatal screening and diagnostic testing, giving women more information to choose from when it comes to their care and treatment options.

Myth 5: Motherhood is unsuitable for women over 40.

This fallacy damages the value of parenthood at any age and reinforces ageist attitudes. In actuality, women in their 40s and beyond are perfectly capable of being devoted, caring parents; there is no upper age limit for parenting. An abundance of wisdom, maturity, and life experience are brought to the parenting journey by older mothers, whether they are growing their current family or starting one for the first time.

Furthermore, studies have indicated that the stability, resources, and emotional maturity that older parents frequently bring to their parenting duties may be advantageous to children born to these moms. Parenting later in life can present certain difficulties, such as controlling energy levels and juggling conflicting objectives, although these obstacles are surmountable with assistance, resiliency, and a robust support system.

Myth 6: Age is the only factor affecting fertility.

When the Fact is Several other factors influence fertility, which includes: Underlying medical conditions can impact both male and female fertility. Lifestyle such as Smoking, excessive alcohol consumption, and poor diet can decrease fertility and Partner's fertility are factor that contributes to infertility in roughly 30% of cases.

Myth 7: Having children later in life means less time with them.

While Fact is There are many fulfilling ways to experience parenthood, and older parents often bring valuable life experience and maturity to raising children.

Finally, dispelling myths and false beliefs about older women's fertility is crucial for enabling women to take charge of their reproductive health, encouraging informed decision-making, and combating ageist attitudes that minimize the significance of parenting at any age. Women may be empowered, resilient, and full of hope as they manage the challenges of fertility after 40 by being given evidence-based knowledge, resources, and support.

The Importance of Mindset and Emotional Well-being in the Fertility Journey

The journey to parenthood is often portrayed as a joyous and fulfilling experience, but for many individuals and couples struggling with infertility, it can be a rollercoaster of emotions fraught with uncertainty, disappointment, and despair. In the midst of medical treatments, diagnostic tests, and fertility interventions, it's easy for individuals to overlook the profound impact that mindset and emotional well-being can have on their fertility journey. However, cultivating a positive mindset and prioritizing emotional well-being are essential components of navigating the challenges of infertility and maximizing the chances of achieving a successful pregnancy. In this discussion, we will explore the importance of mindset and emotional well-being in the fertility journey and offer strategies for maintaining resilience, hope, and positivity in the face of adversity.

1. Acknowledging and Validating Emotions

The first step in prioritizing emotional well-being on the fertility journey is to acknowledge and validate the range of emotions that individuals may experience. From feelings of grief, anger, and frustration to anxiety, guilt, and shame, infertility can evoke a complex array of emotions that can be overwhelming to process. It's important for individuals to give themselves permission to feel and express these emotions without judgment or self-criticism. Seeking support from loved ones, friends, support groups, or mental health professionals can provide a safe space to share experiences, gain perspective, and receive validation for one's feelings.

2. Cultivating Resilience and Optimism

Maintaining resilience and optimism in the face of infertility can be challenging, but it is essential for navigating the ups and downs of the fertility journey. Cultivating resilience involves developing coping skills, such as problem-solving, assertiveness, and emotional regulation, that enable individuals to adapt to adversity and bounce back from setbacks. Strategies such as mindfulness meditation, yoga, journaling, and creative expression can also help individuals manage stress, reduce anxiety, and foster a sense of inner calm and resilience. Additionally, cultivating a sense of optimism and hope can help individuals stay motivated and resilient in the face of uncertainty, setbacks, and disappointments. Setting realistic goals, focusing on what is within one's control, and celebrating small victories along the way can help individuals maintain a positive outlook and stay committed to their fertility journey.

3. Prioritizing Self-care and Well-being

Self-care is essential for maintaining emotional well-being and resilience on the fertility journey. This includes prioritizing activities and practices that nourish the mind, body, and spirit, such as regular exercise, nutritious eating, adequate sleep, and relaxation techniques. Engaging in activities that bring joy, pleasure, and fulfillment can also help individuals maintain a sense of balance and perspective amidst the stress and uncertainty of infertility. Setting boundaries, practicing assertiveness, and saying no to activities or commitments that drain energy or cause distress can help individuals protect their emotional well-being and preserve their mental and physical health.

4. Building a Support Network

Social support is a critical resource for individuals facing infertility, providing emotional validation, practical assistance, and a sense of belonging and connection. Building a support network of friends, family members, support groups, and online communities can help individuals feel less isolated and alone in their fertility journey. Sharing experiences, information, and resources with others who are going through similar challenges can provide validation, empathy, and encouragement.

Additionally, seeking support from mental health professionals, fertility counselors, or spiritual advisors can offer personalized guidance, coping strategies, and emotional support tailored to one's individual needs.

5. Practicing Mindfulness and Acceptance

Mindfulness and acceptance-based approaches can help individuals cultivate a greater sense of peace, acceptance, and resilience in the face of infertility. Mindfulness involves bringing non-judgmental awareness to the present moment, observing thoughts, feelings, and sensations with curiosity and compassion. Acceptance involves acknowledging and making peace with difficult emotions, thoughts, and experiences, rather than resisting or avoiding them. Mindfulness-based practices such as mindfulness meditation, body scan, and mindful movement can help individuals develop greater self-awareness, emotional regulation, and resilience in the face of infertility.

6. Seeking Professional Support

Finally, it's important for individuals struggling with infertility to seek professional support from qualified mental health professionals who specialize in fertility counseling and reproductive psychology. Fertility counselors can provide individualized support, coping strategies, and therapeutic interventions to help individuals navigate the emotional complexities of infertility and make informed decisions about their fertility journey. Additionally, reproductive psychologists can offer psychological assessments, counseling, and support services to individuals and couples undergoing fertility treatments, donor conception, surrogacy, or adoption.

Finally, prioritizing mindset and emotional well-being is essential for individuals navigating the challenges of infertility and maximizing their chances of achieving a successful pregnancy. By acknowledging and validating emotions, cultivating resilience and optimism, prioritizing self-care and well-being, building a support network, practicing mindfulness and acceptance, and seeking professional support when needed, individuals can cultivate greater emotional resilience, hope, and well-being on their fertility journey. Ultimately, by prioritizing emotional well-being and resilience, individuals can navigate the challenges of infertility with greater ease, grace, and resilience, and ultimately achieve their goal of building a family.

Although there is a correlation between maternal age and the likelihood of specific chromosomal disorders, such Down syndrome, the overall risk is still rather low. As opposed to 1 in 1,250 at age 25, the Centers for Disease Control and Prevention (CDC) estimates that the chance of having a child with Down syndrome at age 40 is about 1 in 100.

It's crucial to remember that the great majority of infants born to older moms are healthy and defect-free. Furthermore, chromosomal abnormalities can now be detected early in pregnancy thanks to advancements in prenatal screening and diagnostic testing, giving women more information to choose from when it comes to their care and treatment options.

CHAPTER 2

Nutrition and Lifestyle Optimization in the Fertility Journey

Optimizing nutrition and lifestyle habits is essential for individuals navigating the challenges of infertility and seeking to enhance their fertility potential. A balanced diet rich in nutrient-dense foods such as fruits, vegetables, whole grains, lean proteins, and healthy fats provides essential vitamins, minerals, and antioxidants that support hormonal balance and reproductive health. Adequate hydration, regular physical activity, and stress management techniques such as mindfulness meditation and yoga can further support fertility by promoting hormone regulation, reducing stress levels, and improving overall well-being.

Maintaining a healthy weight is also important for optimizing fertility, as both overweight and underweight individuals may experience disruptions in hormone levels and menstrual irregularities that can affect fertility. Achieving a healthy weight through a balanced diet and regular exercise can help regulate ovulation and enhance fertility potential. Additionally, limiting exposure to environmental toxins and chemicals, such as smoking, alcohol, and pesticides, can help protect fertility and reproductive health.

By prioritizing nutrition and lifestyle optimization, individuals can empower themselves to take an active role in their fertility journey and promote overall health and well-being. Consulting with a healthcare provider or registered dietitian can provide personalized guidance and support for individuals seeking to optimize their fertility through nutrition and lifestyle modifications. Ultimately, making informed choices about diet, exercise, hydration, stress management, and environmental exposures can help individuals maximize their fertility potential and increase their chances of achieving a healthy pregnancy.

The Role of Nutrition in Supporting Fertility and Reproductive Health

Nutrition plays a fundamental role in supporting fertility and reproductive health, influencing various aspects of reproductive function, from hormone production to egg and sperm quality. As individuals navigate the journey to parenthood, making informed choices about diet and nutrition can have a profound impact on fertility outcomes and overall reproductive well-being. In this comprehensive discussion, we will explore the key nutrients, dietary patterns, and lifestyle factors that contribute to optimal fertility and reproductive health, offering evidence-based insights and practical recommendations for individuals seeking to enhance their fertility potential.

1. Essential Nutrients for Fertility

Certain nutrients are particularly important for supporting fertility and reproductive health, playing key roles in hormone regulation, egg and sperm development, and embryo implantation. These nutrients include:

- *Folate:* Folate, also known as vitamin B9, is essential for DNA synthesis and cell division, making it critical for healthy egg and sperm development. Adequate folate intake has been associated with improved fertility outcomes and reduced risk of neural tube defects in pregnancy.

- ***Iron:*** Iron is necessary for oxygen transport, energy metabolism, and cellular function, all of which are important for supporting fertility and reproductive health. Iron deficiency can lead to menstrual irregularities, ovulatory dysfunction, and impaired egg quality.

- ***Omega-3 Fatty Acids:*** Omega-3 fatty acids, particularly EPA and DHA found in fatty fish and seafood, play a crucial role in hormone production, inflammation regulation, and reproductive function. Omega-3 fatty acids have been linked to improved egg quality, embryo development, and pregnancy outcomes.

- ***Antioxidants:*** Antioxidants such as vitamin C, vitamin E, selenium, and zinc help protect reproductive cells from oxidative damage caused by free radicals, which can impair fertility and reproductive health. Antioxidants have been shown to improve sperm quality, reduce DNA damage, and enhance embryo development.

- ***Vitamin D:*** Vitamin D is important for hormone regulation, immune function, and bone health, all of which are relevant to fertility and reproductive health. Low vitamin D levels have been associated with menstrual irregularities, ovulatory dysfunction, and reduced fertility.

- ***Protein:*** Adequate protein intake is essential for supporting reproductive hormone production, egg and sperm development, and embryo implantation. Protein sources such as lean meats, poultry, fish, eggs, dairy products, legumes, and nuts provide essential amino acids and nutrients that support fertility and reproductive health.

2. Dietary Patterns and Fertility

In addition to individual nutrients, overall dietary patterns and food choices can also influence fertility and reproductive health. Research suggests that certain dietary patterns may be more beneficial for fertility than others:

- ***Mediterranean Diet:*** The Mediterranean diet, characterized by high consumption of fruits, vegetables, whole grains, legumes, nuts, seeds, olive oil, and fish, has been associated with improved fertility outcomes in both men and women. This dietary pattern provides a rich array of vitamins, minerals, antioxidants, and healthy fats that support reproductive health.

- ***DASH Diet:*** The Dietary Approaches to Stop Hypertension (DASH) diet, which emphasizes fruits, vegetables, whole grains, lean proteins, and low-fat dairy products while limiting sodium, saturated fats, and refined sugars, has also been linked to improved fertility in women. The DASH diet may help regulate insulin levels, reduce inflammation, and support hormonal balance, all of which are important for fertility.

- ***Plant-Based Diet:*** Plant-based diets rich in fruits, vegetables, whole grains, legumes, nuts, and seeds provide a wealth of nutrients, fiber, and phytonutrients that support fertility and reproductive health. Research suggests that plant-based diets may be associated with improved fertility outcomes and reduced risk of ovulatory infertility.

3. Lifestyle Factors and Fertility

In addition to diet, certain lifestyle factors can also influence fertility and reproductive health:

- ***Maintaining a Healthy Weight:*** Both underweight and overweight individuals may experience fertility challenges, as extremes in weight can disrupt hormone levels, menstrual cycles, and ovulation. Achieving and maintaining a healthy weight through a balanced diet and regular exercise is important for optimizing fertility and reproductive health.

- ***Moderate Exercise:*** Regular physical activity is beneficial for supporting fertility and reproductive health, as it helps regulate hormone levels, reduce stress, and improve circulation. Engaging in moderate-intensity activities such as brisk walking, swimming, cycling, or yoga for at least 30 minutes most days of the week can support fertility and overall well-being.

- ***Avoiding Excessive Alcohol and Caffeine:*** Excessive alcohol consumption and caffeine intake have been associated with reduced fertility and pregnancy outcomes. Limiting alcohol consumption to moderate levels (one drink per day for women) and caffeine intake to 200-300 mg per day (equivalent to 1-2 cups of coffee) may help support fertility and reproductive health.

- ***Avoiding Tobacco and Recreational Drugs:*** Smoking and recreational drug use can have detrimental effects on fertility and reproductive health, affecting hormone levels, sperm quality, and egg quality. Quitting smoking and avoiding recreational drug use are important steps for optimizing fertility and increasing the chances of achieving a healthy pregnancy.

- ***Managing Stress:*** Chronic stress can negatively impact fertility by disrupting hormone balance, affecting ovulation, and reducing sperm quality. Finding healthy ways to manage stress, such as mindfulness meditation, deep breathing exercises, yoga, tai chi, and progressive muscle relaxation, can help individuals reduce stress levels and support reproductive health.

4. Supplements for Fertility

In addition to obtaining nutrients from food sources, some individuals may benefit from taking supplements to support fertility and reproductive health. Common supplements for fertility include:

- ***Folic Acid:*** Folic acid supplementation is recommended for women planning to conceive, as it plays a crucial role in preventing neural tube defects in early pregnancy. Women of childbearing age are advised to take a daily supplement containing 400-800 micrograms of folic acid to support fertility and reduce the risk of birth defects.

- ***Prenatal Vitamins:*** Prenatal vitamins are formulated to provide essential nutrients that support fertility, pregnancy, and fetal development. These supplements typically contain folic acid, iron, calcium, vitamin D, and other vitamins and minerals important for reproductive health. Taking a prenatal vitamin before conception and throughout pregnancy can help ensure that individuals meet their nutritional needs and support optimal fertility and pregnancy outcomes.

- ***Omega-3 Fatty Acids:*** Omega-3 fatty acid supplements, particularly those containing EPA and DHA, may be beneficial for supporting fertility and reproductive health. Fish oil supplements derived from cold-water fatty fish such as salmon, mackerel, and sardines provide EPA and DHA, which have been associated with improved egg quality, embryo development, and pregnancy outcomes.

- ***Coenzyme Q10 (CoQ10):*** Coenzyme Q10 is an antioxidant that plays a critical role in energy production and cellular function. CoQ10 supplementation may help support fertility by improving egg quality, sperm motility, and mitochondrial function. Research suggests that CoQ10 supplementation may be particularly beneficial for individuals of advanced reproductive age or those with age-related fertility decline.

- ***Vitamin D:*** Vitamin D supplementation may be beneficial for individuals with low vitamin D levels, as vitamin D deficiency has been associated with menstrual irregularities, ovulatory dysfunction, and reduced fertility. Taking a vitamin D supplement, particularly during the winter months or for individuals with limited sun exposure, can help support hormonal balance and reproductive health.

- ***Probiotics:*** Probiotic supplements containing beneficial bacteria such as Lactobacillus and Bifidobacterium may support fertility by promoting gut health and immune function. Emerging research suggests that the gut microbiome may play a role in fertility and reproductive health, and probiotic supplementation may help support a healthy gut microbiome and optimize fertility potential.

In summary, nutrition plays a critical role in supporting fertility and reproductive health, influencing various aspects of reproductive function, hormone regulation, and fertility potential. By focusing on a balanced diet rich in essential nutrients, adopting healthy lifestyle habits, and considering supplementation when needed, individuals can optimize their fertility and increase their chances of achieving a healthy pregnancy. Consulting with a healthcare provider or registered dietitian can provide personalized guidance and support for individuals seeking to enhance their fertility through nutrition and lifestyle modifications. Ultimately, prioritizing nutrition and lifestyle optimization can empower individuals to take an active role in their fertility journey and promote overall health and well-being.

Implementing Lifestyle Changes to Enhance Fertility Potential

Embarking on the journey to parenthood can be both exciting and challenging, particularly for individuals facing fertility struggles. While medical interventions such as assisted reproductive technologies (ART) can play a crucial role in overcoming infertility, lifestyle factors also significantly impact fertility potential. Making informed choices and implementing lifestyle changes can optimize fertility outcomes and increase the chances of conceiving naturally or with medical assistance. In this comprehensive discussion, we will explore various lifestyle changes that individuals can implement to enhance their fertility potential, offering evidence-based insights and practical recommendations for promoting reproductive health and well-being.

1. Nutrition and Diet

A balanced and nutritious diet is essential for supporting fertility and reproductive health. Individuals can optimize their fertility potential by focusing on the following dietary recommendations:

- ***Eat a Variety of Nutrient-Dense Foods:*** Incorporate a diverse range of fruits, vegetables, whole grains, lean proteins, and healthy fats into your diet to ensure you're getting a wide array of essential nutrients.

- ***Emphasize Plant-Based Foods:*** Plant-based foods such as fruits, vegetables, legumes, nuts, and seeds are rich in vitamins, minerals, antioxidants, and phytonutrients that support fertility and reproductive health.

- ***Choose Healthy Fats:*** Opt for sources of healthy fats such as avocados, nuts, seeds, olive oil, and fatty fish, which provide omega-3 fatty acids and other essential nutrients that support hormone production and reproductive function.

- ***Limit Processed Foods and Added Sugars:*** Minimize consumption of processed foods, sugary beverages, and foods high in added sugars, as these can contribute to inflammation, hormonal imbalances, and impaired fertility.

- ***Stay Hydrated:*** Drink plenty of water throughout the day to stay hydrated and support overall health and well-being. Limit consumption of caffeinated and alcoholic beverages, which can negatively impact fertility.

2. Weight Management

Sustaining a healthy weight is essential to maximizing the results of conception. Both underweight and overweight individuals may experience fertility challenges, as extremes in weight can disrupt hormone levels, menstrual cycles, and ovulation. Implementing strategies for weight management can help support fertility:

- ***Achieve a Healthy Weight:*** Work with a healthcare provider or registered dietitian to achieve and maintain a healthy weight through a balanced diet and regular exercise. Aim for a body mass index (BMI) within the healthy range (18.5-24.9 kg/m^2).

- ***Regular Physical Activity:*** Engage in regular physical activity to support weight management and overall health. Aim for two or more days of muscle-strengthening exercises per week in addition to at least 150 minutes of moderate-intensity activity or 75 minutes of vigorous-intensity exercise every week..

- ***Monitor Portion Sizes:*** Pay attention to portion sizes and practice mindful eating to avoid overeating and promote healthy weight management. Focus on eating until you're satisfied, rather than overeating or restricting food intake.

3. Exercise and Physical Activity

Regular exercise is beneficial for supporting fertility and reproductive health. Physical activity helps regulate hormone levels, reduce stress, and improve circulation, all of which can contribute to enhanced fertility. Consider the following recommendations for incorporating exercise into your routine:

- *Find Activities You Enjoy:* Choose physical activities that you enjoy and can stick with long term. Whether it's walking, jogging, cycling, swimming, yoga, or dance, find activities that bring you joy and make exercise a regular part of your routine.

- *Mix It Up:* Incorporate a variety of aerobic, strength-training, and flexibility exercises into your routine to support overall fitness and well-being. Mix up your workouts to prevent boredom and challenge different muscle groups.

- ***Be Consistent:*** Aim for consistency in your exercise routine by scheduling regular workouts and making physical activity a priority. Start with manageable goals and gradually increase the duration and intensity of your workouts as you build strength and endurance.

- ***Listen to Your Body:*** Pay attention to your body's cues and adjust your exercise routine as needed. If you're experiencing fatigue, discomfort, or pain, take a break or modify your workouts to avoid injury and promote recovery.

4. Stress Management

Chronic stress can negatively impact fertility by disrupting hormone balance, affecting ovulation, and reducing sperm quality. Implementing stress management techniques can help support fertility and reproductive health:

- ***Practice Mindfulness Meditation:*** Mindfulness meditation involves bringing non-judgmental awareness to the present moment, which can help reduce stress, promote relaxation, and improve emotional well-being.

- ***Deep Breathing Exercises:*** Deep breathing exercises such as diaphragmatic breathing, belly breathing, or box breathing can help activate the body's relaxation response, reduce stress levels, and promote feelings of calm and tranquility.

- ***Yoga and Tai Chi:*** Yoga and tai chi are mind-body practices that combine gentle movements, breathwork, and mindfulness to promote relaxation, reduce stress, and improve flexibility and strength.

- ***Progressive Muscle Relaxation:*** Progressive muscle relaxation involves tensing and relaxing different muscle groups in the body to release tension, reduce stress, and promote physical and mental relaxation.

5. Environmental Exposures

Limiting exposure to environmental toxins and chemicals can help protect fertility and reproductive health. Individuals can take steps to minimize exposure to potential natural dangers and advance a sound regenerative environment:

- ***Maintain a strategic distance from Smoking and Used Smoke:*** Smoking and introduction to used smoke can have inconvenient impacts on richness and regenerative wellbeing, influencing hormone levels, sperm quality, and egg quality. Stopping smoking and maintaining a strategic distance from presentation to used smoke are fundamental for optimizing ripeness results.

- ***Restrain Liquor Utilization:*** Intemperate liquor utilization has been related with decreased richness and pregnancy results. Restrain liquor admissions to direct levels (up to one drink per day for ladies and up to two drinks per day for men) or dodge liquor inside and out when attempting to conceive.

- ***Minimize Presentation to Pesticides and Chemicals:*** Minimize presentation to pesticides, herbicides, and other natural chemicals which will disturb hormone work and regenerative wellbeing. Select natural nourishments when conceivable, and utilize normal and eco-friendly family and individual care items to diminish presentation to destructive chemicals.

- ***Be Cautious with Medicines and Supplements:*** Be cautious with medicines and supplements which will influence ripeness or regenerative wellbeing. Counsel with a healthcare supplier some time recently beginning or ceasing any solutions or supplements, particularly in the event that you're attempting to conceive or experiencing ripeness medicines.

- ***Dodge Intemperate Warm Introduction:*** Delayed introduction to over the top warm, such as hot tubs, saunas, or hot showers, can briefly diminish sperm generation and influence sperm quality. Restrain introduction to intemperate warm and keep up a solid body temperature to bolster ideal sperm generation and ripeness.

6. Rest Cleanliness

Getting satisfactory and quality rest is basic for supporting ripeness and regenerative wellbeing. Destitute rest propensities and rest unsettling influences can disturb hormone levels, influence menstrual cycles, and impede ripeness. Consider the taking after tips for advancing solid sleep hygiene:

- ***Set up a Reliable Rest Plan:*** Go to bed and wake up at the same time each day, indeed on ends of the week, to control your body's inside clock and advance superior rest quality.

- ***Make an Unwinding Sleep time Schedule:*** Build up a unwinding sleep time schedule to flag to your body that it's time to wind down and get ready for rest. Activities such as perusing, taking a warm shower, practicing unwinding methods, or tuning in to calming music can offer assistance advance unwinding and make strides rest quality.

- ***Create a Comfortable Rest Environment:*** Make a sleep-friendly environment that's cool, dull, and calm to advance ideal rest conditions. Contribute in a comfortable sleeping pad and pads, utilize power outage window ornaments or eye veils to piece out light, and utilize white commotion machines or earplugs to square out commotion and diversions.

- ***Constrain Screen Time Some time recently Bed:*** Diminish presentation to electronic gadgets such as smartphones, tablets, computers, and tvs some time recently sleep time, as the blue light transmitted from these gadgets can disturb rest designs and meddled with melatonin generation.

- ***Maintain a strategic distance from Stimulants Some time recently Bed:*** Dodge devouring caffeine, nicotine, and liquor near to sleep time, as these substances can meddled with rest quality and disturb your ability to drop sleeping and remain sleeping.

7. Looking for Proficient Back

In expansion to actualizing way of life changes, people confronting richness challenges may advantage from looking for proficient back and direction. Ripeness masters, regenerative endocrinologists, and richness counsellors can give personalized appraisals, symptomatic testing, and treatment choices custom fitted to person needs. Moreover, back bunches, counselling administrations, and online communities can offer passionate bolster, approval, and support all through the richness travel.

So, Setting out on the travel to parenthood is a deeply individual and transformative involvement, and optimizing richness potential requires a all encompassing approach that addresses different angles of physical, passionate, and natural well-being. By making educated choices and actualizing way of life changes that bolster regenerative wellbeing, people can improve their ripeness potential and increment the probability of accomplishing a sound pregnancy. Whether conceiving actually or with restorative help, prioritizing sustenance, work out, stretch administration, rest cleanliness, and natural wellbeing can enable people to require an dynamic part in their richness travel and develop a strong and sustaining regenerative environment. Seeking proficient bolster, direction, and assets can assist upgrade richness results and give profitable bolster all through the ripeness travel. Eventually, by prioritizing lifestyle changes that advance regenerative wellbeing and well-being, people can set out on their travel to parenthood with certainty, resilience, and good faith for long haul.

Strategies for Managing Stress and Optimizing Overall well-being

Managing the difficulties of infertility can be a difficult emotional journey that is frequently marked by stress, frustration, and uncertainty. To optimize conception outcomes and promote general health, it is imperative to prioritize stress management and overall well-being in addition to the demands of fertility treatments. We will cover a wide range of stress management and overall well-being optimization techniques during the reproductive journey in this in-depth talk. We will provide evidence-based insights and useful suggestions for building emotional health, resilience, and empowerment.

1. Meditation with mindfulness

One of the most effective methods for reducing stress and fostering emotional health is mindfulness meditation. Mindfulness meditation fosters present-moment awareness and acceptance without judgment, which helps people become more resilient, emotionally stable, and peaceful within. Regular mindfulness meditation has been demonstrated to alleviate stress, alleviate depression, anxiety, and enhance mood, quality of sleep, and psychological health in general. Even for a short while each day, practicing mindfulness meditation can help people become more resilient and manage the difficulties associated with infertility.

2. Practices for Deep Breathing

Deep breathing exercises, like box breathing, diaphragmatic breathing, and belly breathing, are easy yet powerful ways to ease tension and encourage calm. By triggering the body's relaxation response, deep breathing helps to lower heart rate, ease tense muscles, and promote mental clarity. Regularly engaging in deep breathing techniques can help people regain equilibrium and serenity, which will make it easier and more resilient for them to manage the reproductive journey—especially during times of increased stress or anxiety.

3. Tai Chi and Yoga

Gentle movements, breathwork, and mindfulness are combined in mind-body activities like yoga and tai chi to enhance general well-being, lower stress levels, and encourage relaxation. The emphasis on body and breath awareness in tai chi and yoga promotes inner calm, connection, and grounding. Regular yoga or tai chi practice has been linked to improved mood, better sleep, improved physical function, and a reduction in stress, anxiety, and depression, according to research. Adding yoga or tai chi to your practice can be a great way to relax, rejuvenate, and take care of your body and mind while dealing with the challenges of infertility.

4. Gradual Release of Tensed Muscles

A relaxation technique called progressive muscular relaxation includes tensing and relaxing various muscle groups in the body to lessen stress, ease tension, and encourage both mental and physical relaxation. Progressive muscle relaxation helps people become more aware of and release tension contained in the body by methodically tensing and relaxing different muscular groups. This promotes a profound sense of relaxation and well-being. Progressive muscle relaxation is a regular exercise that can help people sleep better, manage stress more successfully, and generally improve their physical and mental well-being.

5. Keeping a Journal and Expressing Yourself

During the fertility journey, journaling and artistic expression are useful methods for getting clarity, processing emotions, and promoting self-expression. Maintaining a journal gives people a private, safe environment to examine their ideas, emotions, and experiences. It also serves as a tool for introspection and emotional release. Likewise, partaking in artistic endeavors such Activities that allow people to express themselves creatively, connect with their inner wisdom, and find purpose and comfort in the face of infertility include writing, painting, drawing, and creating. Including journaling and artistic expression in your daily routine can offer a healing way to process feelings, lower stress levels, and enhance general wellbeing.

6. Seeking Assistance

It is crucial to ask for help from friends, family, support groups, or mental health specialists in order to manage stress and foster emotional wellbeing while going through the reproductive process. Sharing ideas, feelings, and experiences with others you can trust can offer support, empathy, and validation, making people feel less alone and isolated in their challenges. A sense of community and belonging can be gained by joining an online community or fertility support group, which can also provide helpful resources, information, and support from people facing comparable difficulties. In addition, getting help from a mental health specialist or fertility counselor can help you manage the emotional complexities of infertility with more resilience and self-awareness by offering you individualized guidance, coping mechanisms, and emotional support catered to your particular needs.

7. Techniques for Self-Care

Making self-care a priority is crucial for stress management, mental health promotion, and maintaining general well-being and happiness during the reproductive process. A vast array of practices and activities that support the mind, body, and spirit are included in self-care. These include:

- ***Healthy Lifestyle Habits:*** Make physical health and wellbeing a priority by giving regular exercise, a balanced diet, enough sleep, and relaxation techniques top priority.

- ***Setting Boundaries:*** To safeguard your emotional well-being and maintain your physical and mental health, set clear boundaries around your time, energy, and resources.

- ***Making Time for Pleasurable Activities:*** Whether it's hanging out with loved ones, pursuing interests and hobbies, or taking in the scenery and outdoors, schedule time for activities that make you happy, content, and fulfilled.

- ***How to Exercise Self-Compassion:*** Treat yourself with kindness and compassion, especially when things are hard. Show yourself the same consideration, tolerance, and acceptance that you would show a close friend or family member.

- ***Seeking Joy and Gratitude:*** No matter how tiny, learn to be grateful and appreciative of the joys and gifts in your life. Amidst the difficulties of infertility, keep your attention on the here and now and look for happy and beautiful moments. During the reproductive journey, you can maintain your general well-being, lower stress levels, and regain your energy by implementing these self-care routines into your routine.

In summary, Navigating the obstacles of infertility and maximizing reproductive potential require controlling stress and improving general well-being. You can cultivate greater resilience, emotional well-being, and empowerment on your fertility journey by adding mindfulness meditation, deep breathing exercises, yoga and tai chi, progressive muscle relaxation, journaling and creative expression, seeking support, and making self-care practices a priority into your routine. Remind yourself that taking care of yourself is not selfish; rather, it is an important investment in your physical, mental, and emotional well-being that will enable you to handle the ups and downs of infertility with fortitude, grace, and courage.

CHAPTER 3

Cutting-Edge Fertility Technologies

In recent decades, remarkable advancements in wisdom and technology have converted the geography of fertility treatment, offering new stopgap and possibilities for individualities and couples floundering to conceive. These slice-edge fertility technologies harness the power of invention to address colorful causes of gravidity and ameliorate the chances of successful generality. From groundbreaking procedures to sophisticated laboratory ways, these advancements have revolutionized the field of reproductive drug, furnishing unknown openings for individualities to make their families.

In this period of rapid-fire technological progress, the boundaries of what was formerly supposed possible in fertility treatment are continually being pushed and expanded. The preface of new ways and procedures has not only enhanced the success rates of supported reproductive technologies but has also paved the way for further substantiated and acclimatized approaches to fertility care. As a result, individualities facing gravidity now have access to a different array of slice- edge treatments and interventions designed to address their unique requirements and circumstances.

This comprehensive disquisition will claw into the world of slice- edge fertility technologies, examining the rearmost advancements and inventions shaping the field of reproductive drug. From in vitro fertilization (IVF) with preimplantation inheritable testing to artificial intelligence (AI) and prophetic analytics, each technology offers new openings for individualities to overcome fertility challenges and realize their dreams of parenting. By understanding the capabilities and eventuality of these slice- edge fertility technologies, individualities and couples can make informed opinions about their fertility care trip, empowered by the knowledge that groundbreaking results are within reach.

Overview of Modern Fertility Treatments and Technologies for Women Over 40

As women detention travail for colorful particular, professional, and social reasons, the demand for fertility treatments and technologies among women over 40 has grown significantly in recent times. Advances in reproductive drug have expanded the options available to women seeking to conceive latterly in life, offering innovative treatments and technologies designed to address age- related fertility challenges. From supported reproductive technologies to slice- edge interventions, this overview provides a comprehensive examination of ultramodern fertility treatments and technologies available for women over 40.

1. Supported Reproductive Technologies(ART)

Supported reproductive technologies(ART) encompass a range of fertility treatments designed to help individualities and couples in achieving gestation when natural generality isn't successful. Some of the most common ART options available to women over 40 include

- ***In Vitro Fertilization (IVF)*** IVF involves the fertilization of eggs with sperm in a laboratory setting, followed by the transfer of performing embryos into the uterus. IVF can be particularly salutary for women over

40 who may witness age-affiliated declines in egg quality and volume.

- ***Intracytoplasmic Sperm Injection (ICSI):*** ICSI is a technical form of IVF where a single sperm is fitted directly into an egg to grease fertilization. This fashion can be used to overcome manly factor gravidity or to ameliorate fertilization rates in cases of advanced motherly age.

- ***Preimplantation inheritable Testing (PGT):*** PGT involves webbing embryos for inheritable abnormalities before implantation, allowing for the selection of embryos with the loftiest liability of implantation and healthy development. PGT can be particularly precious for women over 40, who may be at increased threat of chromosomal abnormalities and confinement.

2. Oocyte Cryopreservation (Egg Indurating)

Oocyte cryopreservation, or egg freezing, has surfaced as a precious option for women over 40 who wish to save their fertility for unborn use. This fashion involves reacquiring and indurating a woman's eggs for after use, allowing her to delay travail while conserving her fertility eventuality. Egg freezing can be particularly salutary for women who aren't yet ready to start a family but wish to retain the option for unborn gestation.

3. Donor Egg IVF

For women over 40 who witness age-affiliated declines in egg quality or volume, patron egg IVF may offer a pathway to gestation. This involves using eggs bestowed by a youngish woman, generally in her 20s or 30s, to achieve fertilization through IVF. patron egg IVF can be largely successful in helping women over 40 conceive and carry a gestation to term, as it circumvents age-related egg quality issues.

4. Ovarian revivification remedy

Ovarian revivification remedy is a slice- edge fertility treatment that aims to stimulate ovarian function and ameliorate egg quality in women over 40. This innovative fashion involves using stem cells, growth factors, or platelet-rich tube(PRP) to rejuvenate the ovaries and enhance fertility eventuality. While still considered experimental, ovarian revivification remedy holds pledge as a implicit option for women seeking to ameliorate their chances of generality latterly in life.

5. Natural Cycle IVF

Natural cycle IVF is an indispensable approach to traditional IVF that involves retrieving and fertilizing a woman's naturally ovulated egg without the use of ovarian stimulation medicines. This approach may be particularly suitable for women over 40 who prefer a more natural and minimally invasive fertility treatment option. Natural cycle IVF may offer advantages similar as reduced drug burden and lower treatment costs, although success rates may vary compared to conventional IVF.

6. Advanced Reproductive ways

In addition to traditional ART options, ongoing exploration and development in the field of reproductive drug continue to yield innovative ways and interventions for women over 40. These advanced reproductive ways may include

- ***Mitochondrial relief remedy:*** Mitochondrial relief remedy involves replacing imperfect mitochondria in eggs with healthy mitochondria from a patron egg to help the transmission of mitochondrial conditions and ameliorate fertility eventuality.

- ***Endometrial Receptivity Analysis (period):*** Period is an individual test that assesses the receptivity of the uterine filling to embryo implantation, helping to identify the optimal timing for embryo transfer and ameliorate the chances of successful gestation.

- ***Artificial Intelligence (AI) and Prophetic Analytics:*** AI and prophetic analytics are decreasingly being employed in fertility conventions to dissect large datasets, optimize treatment protocols, and prognosticate the liability of success for individual cases. These technologies may help ameliorate treatment issues and epitomize fertility care for women over 40.

So, the geography of ultramodern fertility treatments and technologies for women over 40 is vast and continually evolving, offering a range of options to address age- related fertility challenges and help individualities achieve their family-structure pretensions. From traditional ART procedures similar as IVF and patron egg IVF to innovative interventions like ovarian revivification remedy and natural cycle IVF, women over 40 have access to a different array of fertility treatments acclimatized to their unique requirements and circumstances. As exploration and technology continue to advance, the future holds indeed lesser pledge for women seeking to conceive latterly in life, with ongoing sweats concentrated on perfecting treatment issues, enhancing patient experience, and expanding access to fertility care.

Exploring Options for Fertility IVF, Egg indurating, and Donor Options

As women detention travail for colorful particular, professional, and social reasons, exploring fertility options becomes decreasingly applicable, especially for those over 40. Advances in reproductive drug have expanded the range of options available, offering stopgap and possibilities for individualities seeking to conceive latterly in life. Among the most prominent options are in vitro fertilization (IVF), egg freezing, and colorful patron options. This comprehensive discussion will explore each option in detail, considering their benefits, considerations, and counteraccusations for women over 40.

1. In Vitro Fertilization (IVF)

In vitro fertilization (IVF) is maybe the most well- known and extensively used supported reproductive technology (ART) for prostrating gravidity. IVF involves the fertilization of eggs with sperm in a laboratory setting, followed by the transfer of performing embryos into the uterus. This fashion offers several advantages for women over 40

- ***Prostrating Age- related Declines:*** IVF can help overcome age-affiliated declines in fertility by bypassing implicit issues with egg quality and volume. With IVF, aged women have the occasion to conceive using their own eggs or, if necessary, patron eggs.

- ***Preimplantation inheritable Testing (PGT):*** For women over 40 who may be at increased threat of chromosomal abnormalities and confinement, IVF with preimplantation inheritable testing (PGT) offers a way to screen embryos for inheritable blights before implantation, adding the chances of a successful gestation.

- ***Individualized Treatment:*** IVF treatment can be acclimatized to individual requirements, with options similar as ICSI(Intracytoplasmic Sperm Injection) available to address manly factor gravidity or egg quality enterprises.

Still, there are considerations and challenges associated with IVF for women over 40

- ***Reduced Success Rates:*** As women age, the success rates of IVF decline due to factors similar as dropped egg quality, lower ovarian reserve, and increased threat of gestation complications. Women over 40 may bear multiple IVF cycles to achieve a successful gestation, and success rates may vary depending on individual circumstances.

- ***Increased pitfalls:*** Aged women witnessing IVF may face increased pitfalls of gestation complications, including gravid diabetes, hypertension, and preterm birth. It's essential for women over 40 considering IVF to bandy these pitfalls with their healthcare providers and make informed opinions about their fertility treatment.

2. Egg indurating

Egg freezing, also known as oocyte cryopreservation, has surfaced as a precious option for women over 40 who wish to save their fertility for unborn use. This fashion involves reacquiring and indurating a woman's eggs for after use, allowing her to delay travail while conserving her fertility eventuality. Egg indurating offers several benefits for women over 40.

- ***Preservation of Fertility:*** Egg indurating allows women to save their fertility while they concentrate on other precedence, similar as career advancement, education, or chancing a suitable mate. By indurating their eggs at a youngish age, women can potentially increase their chances of conceiving latterly in life.

- ***Inflexibility and Control:*** Egg indurating gives women the inflexibility to pursue their reproductive pretensions on their own timeline, without feeling pressured by age- related fertility declines. It provides a sense of control over their reproductive future and allows for further informed decision- making about when to start a family. still, there are considerations and limitations to be apprehensive of with egg freezing.

- ***Age and Egg Quality:*** The success of egg freezing is told by a woman's age at the time of egg reclamation, as youngish women tend to have advanced- quality eggs with better chances of survival after deliquescing. Women over 40 may have smaller feasible eggs available for indurating, and success rates may be lower compared to youngish women.

- ***Cost and Availability:*** Egg freezing can be precious, with costs associated with the original egg reclamation procedure, storehouse freights, and unborn IVF cycles for embryo transfer. also, not all fertility conventions offer egg freezing services, and insurance content may be limited, making it inapproachable for some women over 40.

3. Donor Options

For women over 40 who may witness age-affiliated declines in egg quality or volume, patron options similar as patron eggs or patron embryos offer indispensable pathways to gestation. These options involve using eggs or embryos bestowed by youngish, healthy individualities to achieve fertilization and gestation. patron options give several advantages for women over 40

- ***Prostrating Age- related Challenges:*** Donor eggs or embryos can help overcome age-affiliated declines in egg quality and volume, adding the chances of successful fertilization and gestation for women over 40.

- ***Improved Success Rates:*** Donor options frequently affect in advanced success rates compared to using a woman's own eggs, particularly for women over 40 who may face age- related fertility challenges.

- ***Inheritable Webbing:*** Donor eggs and embryos suffer rigorous webbing for inheritable and chromosomal abnormalities, reducing the threat of inherited inheritable diseases and confinement. still, there are considerations and ethical counteraccusations to be apprehensive of with patron options

- ***Emotional and Cerebral Impact:*** Choosing patron options can raise complex emotional and cerebral issues for intended parents, including passions of grief, loss, and identity enterprises. It's essential for individualities and couples considering patron options to seek comforting and support to address these challenges.

- ***Disclosure and Family Dynamics:*** Intended parents may face opinions about whether and how to expose the use of patron eggs or embryos to their children and extended family members. Open and honest communication about patron generality can help navigate family dynamics and promote understanding and acceptance.

- ***Legal and Ethical Considerations:*** Donor options raise legal and ethical considerations related to concurrence, obscurity, and the rights of benefactors, donors, and performing children. It's important for intended parents to understand and misbehave with applicable laws and guidelines governing patron generality.

To sum it up, exploring options similar as IVF, egg freezing, and patron options can give precious pathways to gestation for women over 40 facing age- related fertility challenges. Each option offers its own benefits, considerations, and counteraccusations , and it's essential for women and their healthcare providers to precisely estimate and bandy the stylish course of action grounded on individual circumstances and preferences. By understanding the range of options available and making informed opinions about fertility treatment, women over 40 can increase their chances of achieving their family- structure pretensions and realizing their dreams of parenting.

Understand the Benefits, Risks, and Considerations Associated with Fertility Treatment styles for Women Over 40

As women detention travail for colorful reasons, fertility treatment styles have come decreasingly applicable, particularly for those over 40 facing age- related fertility challenges. Each system, whether it's in vitro fertilization(IVF), egg freezing, or patron options, comes with its own set of benefits, pitfalls, and considerations. Understanding these factors is pivotal for women and couples as they navigate their fertility trip and make informed opinions about their reproductive options.

1. In Vitro Fertilization (IVF)

Benefits :

- *Prostrating Age- related Fertility Declines:* IVF can help overcome age-affiliated declines in fertility by bypassing implicit issues with egg quality and volume. This is particularly salutary for women over 40 who may witness dropped ovarian reserve and reduced egg quality.

- *Preimplantation inheritable Testing (PGT):* For women over 40 who may be at increased threat of chromosomal abnormalities and confinement, IVF with preimplantation inheritable testing(PGT) offers the occasion to screen embryos for inheritable blights before implantation. This can increase the chances of a successful gestation and reduce the threat of confinement.

- *Individualized Treatment:* IVF treatment can be acclimatized to individual requirements, with options similar as Intracytoplasmic Sperm Injection(ICSI) available to address manly factor gravidity or egg quality enterprises. This substantiated approach allows for the optimization of treatment protocols to maximize success rates.

Risk:

- *Reduced Success Rates:* As women age, the success rates of IVF decline due to factors similar as dropped egg quality, lower ovarian reserve, and increased threat of gestation complications. Women over 40 may bear multiple IVF cycles to achieve a successful gestation, and success rates may vary depending on individual circumstances.

- *Increased risk:* Aged women witnessing IVF may face increased pitfalls of gestation complications, including gravid diabetes, hypertension, and preterm birth. It's essential for women over 40 considering IVF to bandy these pitfalls with their healthcare providers and make informed opinions about their fertility treatment.

Considerations :

- ***lfiscal Costs:*** IVF treatment can be precious, with costs associated with procedures similar as egg reclamation, embryo transfer, specifics, and monitoring. Insurance content for IVF varies, and out-of- fund charges can be significant for women over 40 witnessing multiple cycles of treatment.

- ***Emotional and Cerebral Impact:*** The emotional risk of IVF treatment can be significant, particularly for women over 40 who may face challenges similar as failed cycles, gestation loss, and query about the outgrowth. It's essential for women and couples to seek emotional support and comforting to manage with the stress and anxiety associated with fertility treatment.

2. Egg indurating

Benefits:

- *Preservation of Fertility:* Egg indurating allows women to save their fertility while they concentrate on other precedence, similar as career advancement, education, or chancing a suitable mate. By indurating their eggs at a youngish age, women can potentially increase their chances of conceiving latterly in life.

- *Inflexibility and Control:* Egg indurating gives women the inflexibility to pursue their reproductive pretensions on their own timeline, without feeling pressured by age- related fertility declines. It provides a sense of control over their reproductive future and allows for further informed decision- making about when to start a family.

Risks :

- *Age and Egg Quality:* The success of egg freezing is told by a woman's age at the time of egg reclamation, as youngish women tend to have advanced- quality eggs with better chances of survival after deliquescing. Women over 40 may have smaller feasible eggs available for indurating, and success rates may be lower compared to youngish women.

- *Cost and Availability:* Egg freezing can be precious, with costs associated with the original egg reclamation procedure, storehouse freights, and unborn IVF cycles for embryo transfer. also, not all fertility conventions offer egg freezing services, and insurance content may be limited, making it inapproachable for some women over 40.

Considerations :

- *Timing of Egg indurating :* The optimal age for egg freezing is generally in a woman's 20s or early 30s when egg quality and volume are at their peak. still, numerous women may not consider egg freezing until latterly in life, making it important to weigh the implicit benefits and limitations of the procedure grounded on individual circumstances.

- *Storehouse and Conservation:* Eggs firmed through egg freezing must be stored and maintained at a fertility clinic or cryopreservation installation until they're ready for use. Women over 40 considering egg freezing should consider the long- term storehouse costs and logistics associated with storing their eggs for an extended period.

3. Donor Options

Benefits :

- *Prostrating Age- related Challenges:* Donor options similar as patron eggs or embryos can help overcome age-affiliated declines in egg quality and volume, adding the chances of successful fertilization and gestation for women over 40.

- *Improved Success Rates:* Donor options frequently affect in advanced success rates compared to using a woman's own eggs, particularly for women over 40 who may face age- related fertility challenges.

Risk

- *Emotional and Cerebral Impact:* Choosing patron options can raise complex emotional and cerebral issues for intended parents, including passions of grief, loss, and identity enterprises. It's essential for individualities and couples considering patron options to seek comforting and support to address these challenges.

- *Disclosure and Family Dynamics :* Intended parents may face opinions about whether and how to expose the use of patron eggs or embryos to their children and extended family members. Open and honest communication about patron generality can help navigate family dynamics and promote understanding and acceptance.

Considerations

- *Legal and Ethical Considerations:* Donor options raise legal and ethical considerations related to concurrence, obscurity, and the rights of benefactors, donors, and performing children. It's important for intended parents to understand and misbehave with applicable laws and guidelines governing patron generality.

- *Matching Process:* The process of opting a patron and matching with patron eggs or embryos involves considerations similar as physical characteristics, medical history, and particular preferences. It's important for intended parents to precisely consider these factors and communicate their preferences with their fertility clinic to insure a suitable match.

4. Embryo Adoption

Benefits:

- *Higher Success Rates:* Embryo adoption offers higher success rates compared to traditional IVF using a woman's own eggs, as the embryos are typically of high quality and have been screened for genetic abnormalities.

- *Shared Genetics:* With embryo adoption, intended parents have the opportunity to experience pregnancy and childbirth while sharing a genetic connection with their child, albeit through the donor embryo.

Risks:

- *Emotional Considerations:* Embryo adoption can raise complex emotional considerations for intended parents, including feelings of grief, loss, and identity concerns. It's essential for individuals and couples considering embryo adoption to seek counseling and support to navigate these challenges.

- *Disclosure:* Intended parents may face decisions about whether and how to disclose the use of donor embryos to their children and extended family members. Open and honest communication about embryo adoption can help foster understanding and acceptance within the family.

Considerations:

- *Legal and Ethical Considerations:* Embryo adoption raises legal and ethical considerations related to consent, parental rights, and the rights of donors, recipients, and resulting children. It's important for intended parents to understand and comply with relevant laws and guidelines governing embryo adoption.

- *Matching Process:* The process of matching with donor embryos involves considerations such as physical characteristics, medical history, and personal preferences. Intended parents should communicate their preferences with their fertility clinic and carefully consider their options to ensure a suitable match.

5. Surrogacy

Benefits:

- *Option for Gestational Carriers:* Surrogacy offers an option for women over 40 who are unable to carry a pregnancy themselves due to medical reasons such as uterine abnormalities, recurrent miscarriage, or medical conditions that make pregnancy risky.

- *Genetic Connection:* With gestational surrogacy, intended parents have the opportunity to share a genetic connection with their child, as the embryo is created using the intended mother's eggs or donor eggs and the intended father's sperm.

Risks:

- *Legal and Financial Considerations:* Surrogacy involves complex legal and financial considerations, including contracts, agreements, compensation for the surrogate, and potential legal issues related to parental rights and custody. Intended parents should seek legal counsel and guidance to navigate these complexities.

- *Emotional Considerations:* Surrogacy can raise emotional considerations for all parties involved, including the intended parents, the surrogate, and the resulting child. Open and honest communication, as well as counseling and support, are essential to address these emotional challenges.

Considerations:

- *Matching Process:* The process of matching with a gestational carrier involves considerations such as compatibility, personal preferences, and medical history. Intended parents should work closely with a surrogacy agency or fertility clinic to find a suitable match and establish a supportive relationship with their surrogate.

- *Support and Communication:* Establishing clear communication and support systems with the gestational carrier is essential throughout the surrogacy journey. Intended parents should maintain open communication, show appreciation for the surrogate's role, and provide emotional support throughout the process.

Finally, exploring options such as embryo adoption and surrogacy can provide additional pathways to pregnancy for women over 40 facing age-related fertility challenges. Each method offers its own unique benefits, risks, and considerations that should be carefully evaluated based on individual circumstances, preferences, and values. By thoroughly understanding the potential benefits, risks, and considerations associated with each method, women over 40 can make informed decisions about their fertility journey and choose the path that best aligns with their needs and goals. Additionally, seeking guidance from fertility specialists, counselors, and support networks can provide valuable assistance and support throughout the decision-making process and the fertility treatment journey.

CHAPTER 4

Holistic Approaches to Fertility Enhancement

Holistic methods of enhancing fertility have become more and more popular in recent years as people look for all-encompassing and integrative ways to maximize their chances of getting pregnant. Holistic approaches to medicine acknowledge the connection between mind, body, and spirit in the pursuit of fertility, in contrast to conventional medical treatments that only concentrate on reproductive physiology. Holistic fertility enhancement provides a comprehensive strategy for enhancing fertility and general well-being by addressing the lifestyle, mental, and physical aspects that affect reproductive health.

The underlying principle of holistic fertility enhancement is the understanding that a variety of factors, such as lifestyle choices, emotional health, diet, and environmental conditions, all have an impact on fertility. Holistic approaches recognize the significant influence of stress, nutrition, physical activity, and mental well-being on reproductive function, as opposed to considering fertility as just a physiological process. Individuals and couples can provide the ideal conditions for conception and pregnancy by simultaneously tending to their body, mind, and soul.

A vast array of methods and approaches are included in holistic fertility improvement, such as diet, lifestyle changes, mind-body practices, herbal therapies, and conventional medical modalities. These methods seek to improve sperm health, boost egg quality, help hormonal balance, and advance overall reproductive wellness. Holistic techniques give those with infertility a sense of agency, empowerment, and optimism by enabling them to actively participate in their reproductive journey.

We will delve into the essential elements of holistic fertility care, examine evidence-based practices and interventions, and talk about how individuals and couples can incorporate these approaches into their reproductive journeys in this in-depth examination of holistic approaches to fertility enhancement. We will reveal the intricate network of interrelated variables that affect fertility and the game-changing possibilities of adopting a holistic perspective on reproductive health and well-being through the lens of holistics.

Navigating the Journey of Holistic Practices for Fertility After 40

For numerous women over 40, the desire for parenting remains strong, yet navigating the fertility trip can feel daunting. While conventional medical interventions play a pivotal part, decreasingly, women are turning to holistic practices to round their sweats, seeking a more comprehensive approach to optimize their chances of generality and cultivate emotional well- being throughout the process. This composition explores the implicit benefits of incorporating practices like acupuncture, yoga, and contemplation into fertility care for women above 40.

Understanding Fertility After 40

The natural changes associated with aging can impact fertility. Egg quality and volume decline naturally after 40, making generality more grueling. still, it's pivotal to flash back that gestation after 40 is possible, and numerous women successfully conceive naturally or with supported reproductive technologies (ART) Holistic Practices Beyond the Physical

Holistic practices address the mind- body connection, feting the influence of stress, feelings, and overall well- being on fertility. These practices can round traditional medical interventions by

Reducing stress habitual stress can disrupt hormone regulation and ovulation. Practices like acupuncture, yoga, and contemplation can promote relaxation and stress operation, creating a more conducive terrain for generality.

Improving sleep quality Acceptable sleep is essential for hormonal balance and overall health. These practices can promote better sleep patterns, leading to bettered energy situations and stress adaptability.

Boosting emotional well- being Fertility peregrinations can be emotionally grueling . These practices can help manage anxiety, depression, and negativity, fostering a more positive and empowering mindset.

Exploring the Power of Three

1. Acupuncture: This traditional Chinese drug practice involves fitting thin needles into specific points on the body. Studies suggest acupuncture may regulate hormones, ameliorate blood inflow to the reproductive organs, and reduce stress, potentially enhancing fertility issues.

2. Yoga: Gentle yoga postures and breathing exercises can promote relaxation, reduce stress hormones, and ameliorate rotation. Specific yoga practices may target the pelvic bottom muscles, potentially enhancing uterine health.

3. *Meditation:* Contemplation awareness contemplation fosters present- moment mindfulness and emotional regulation. By quieting the mind and calming the nervous system, contemplation can reduce stress and anxiety, creating a more balanced internal terrain for generality.

Beyond the Individual Practices

Be aware that Eating Nourishing your body with a balanced diet rich in fruits, vegetables, whole grains, and spare protein provides essential nutrients for optimal reproductive health.

Supplements Consulting a healthcare professional about incorporating antenatal vitamins or specific supplements like omega- 3 adipose acids or CoQ10 can be salutary.

erecting a Support Network girding yourself with probative loved bones , musketeers, or joining a fertility support group can give emotional strength and precious participated gests .

Chancing the Right Fit

When incorporating holistic practices, it's important to choose good interpreters and knitter the approach to your individual requirements and preferences. Consider consulting a certified acupuncturist, certified yoga educator endured in fertility, or a meditation teacher specializing in awareness- grounded stress reduction.

Research and resources

While exploration on the specific benefits of these practices for fertility after 40 is ongoing, numerous studies suggest positive impacts on stress operation, emotional well- being, and overall health. Consulting with your healthcare provider and probing estimable sources can help you make informed opinions.

Remember

Holistic practices aren't a cover for conventional medical care. They offer reciprocal support and empower you to take an active part in your fertility trip. For women over 40 navigating the fertility trip, incorporating holistic practices like acupuncture, yoga, and contemplation can offer precious tools for managing stress, enhancing emotional well- being, and creating a more probative terrain for generality. Flash back, your individual requirements and preferences are consummate. By exploring these practices with an open mind and seeking professional guidance, you can empower yourself for a further holistic and positive trip towards achieving your parenting dreams.

Exploring Alternative Therapies and their potential Impact on Fertility

Alternative therapies have garnered increasing attention as supplementary methods to traditional fertility treatments in recent years. The term "alternative therapies" refers to a wide range of non-mainstream medical procedures and methods, such as acupuncture, herbal medicine, chiropractic adjustments, naturopathy, and mind-body therapies. Many people and couples choose alternative therapies as supplemental treatments to aid in their fertility journey, even though the scientific evidence for these therapies' effectiveness in enhancing reproductive outcomes differs.

In this investigation, we will look at some of the most popular alternative treatments for enhancing fertility, investigate possible mechanisms of action, and evaluate the effects of these treatments on fertility based on the available data.

1. Acupuncture:

Acupuncture is a traditional Chinese medicine that stimulates energy flow and restores balance by inserting tiny needles into certain body sites. Acupuncture is frequently used in the context of fertility to support general reproductive health, lessen stress, increase ovarian function, enhance blood flow to the uterus and ovaries, and control monthly cycles. Although the precise processes by which acupuncture affects fertility remain unclear, several studies indicate that treatment may help control hormone levels, promote ovarian function, and lower inflammation—all of which can lead to increased fertility.

There have been conflicting findings from a number of clinical trials looking into how acupuncture affects fertility outcomes. While some studies have revealed no discernible difference between acupuncture treatment groups and control groups, others have documented positive effects of acupuncture on pregnancy rates among women undergoing intrauterine insemination (IUI) or in vitro fertilization (IVF). Many fertility clinics provide acupuncture as a supplemental therapy to traditional therapies despite the variable results, noting its potential benefits for encouraging relaxation, lowering stress levels, and improving overall well-being throughout the reproductive process.

2. Herbal Medicine:

Using substances derived from plants to promote health and cure a range of medical disorders is known as herbal medicine, often referred to as botanical medicine or phytotherapy.

Herbal medicine refers to a broad spectrum of plants and botanical extracts that are thought to improve reproductive health when it comes to fertility. Vitex (chaste tree), maca root, red clover, black cohosh, dong quai, and ginseng are among the common herbs used to increase fertility.

Certain herbs, according to proponents of herbal medicine for conception, can help maintain hormonal balance, control menstrual cycles, improve egg quality, increase sperm motility and production, and lessen inflammation. However, there is little scientific proof of the effectiveness and safety of herbal medication for fertility, therefore using herbal therapies should be done so with caution, especially in female patients using IVF or IUI therapies for fertility. It is crucial that people speak with a trained healthcare professional before utilizing herbal therapies for enhancing fertility because some herbs may interact negatively with pharmaceuticals or have negative effects on reproductive function.

3. Mind-Body Techniques:

Mind-body techniques are a broad category of activities that emphasize how the mind and body are connected in order to enhance health and wellbeing. These methods, which include guided imagery, yoga, meditation, mindfulness, and relaxation exercises, are frequently used to lower stress, anxiety, and depression—all of which have a detrimental effect on fertility. It is thought that mind-body methods help to generate an atmosphere that is conducive to conception and pregnancy by encouraging feelings of calm, relaxation, and inner peace.

Studies have indicated that stress can significantly disrupt menstrual cycles, ovulation, sperm quality, and hormone levels, all of which are related to reproductive health. Throughout the reproductive journey, mind-body therapies provide an all-encompassing approach to stress management and emotional well-being promotion. Numerous studies have shown the potential advantages of mind-body therapies for enhancing the results of fertility, such as higher pregnancy rates, shorter gestational ages, and better mental health.

Chiropractic Care:

A type of complementary and alternative medicine, chiropractic care specializes in the diagnosis and treatment of musculoskeletal conditions, especially those that impact the spine and nervous system. Although there is no scientific evidence linking chiropractic care to enhanced fertility, some chiropractors provide specific treatments targeted at enhancing pelvic alignment and function to improve reproductive health. Chiropractic adjustments have the potential to enhance fertility by regulating nerve function, improving blood flow to the reproductive organs, and correcting poor pelvic alignment.

There is little empirical proof to support the effectiveness of chiropractic care in enhancing fertility, despite the increased interest in this field. There is a dearth of evidence on the effects of chiropractic adjustments on reproductive outcomes, and what is known is not very clear. While some women say that receiving chiropractic treatments has improved their ovulation, fertility, and monthly flow regularly, after receiving chiropractic adjustments; nevertheless, more thorough research is required to support these assertions and demonstrate the security and effectiveness of chiropractic care for enhancing fertility.

Therefore, Alternative therapies offer a holistic approach to fertility enhancement, addressing the physical, emotional, and lifestyle factors that influence reproductive health. While the scientific evidence supporting the efficacy of these therapies varies, many individuals and couples turn to alternative treatments as adjunctive therapies to support their fertility journey. Acupuncture, herbal medicine, mind-body techniques, and chiropractic care are among the most widely used alternative therapies for fertility enhancement, each offering unique benefits and considerations.

While some studies have shown positive effects of alternative therapies on fertility outcomes, more research is needed to fully understand their mechanisms of action and establish their effectiveness as standalone or adjunctive treatments for infertility. Additionally, it's essential for individuals considering alternative therapies to consult with qualified healthcare providers and practitioners, particularly when undergoing fertility treatments such as IVF or IUI. By taking a comprehensive and integrative approach to fertility enhancement, individuals and couples can optimize their chances of conception and create a supportive environment for a healthy pregnancy and childbirth.

Importance of Holistic Approach in Addressing Emotional Issues Concerned with Fertility

The importance of a holistic approach in addressing mind, body, and spirit cannot be overstated, especially in the context of fertility enhancement. Fertility is not solely a physiological process but is influenced by a multitude of factors, including emotional well-being, lifestyle habits, environmental influences, and spiritual beliefs. By addressing the interconnected aspects of mind, body, and spirit, a holistic approach to fertility enhancement recognizes the complex interplay between these elements and seeks to create a supportive environment for conception and pregnancy.

1. Mind:

The mind plays a significant role in fertility, as stress, anxiety, and negative emotions can impact hormone levels, menstrual cycles, ovulation, and sperm quality. By incorporating mind-body techniques such as meditation, mindfulness, yoga, and relaxation exercises, individuals can reduce stress, promote emotional well-being, and create a sense of calm and balance during the fertility journey. These practices not only support mental health but also help cultivate a positive mindset and resilience in the face of challenges.

2. Body:

The body's physical health and wellness are essential factors in fertility. Nutrition, exercise, sleep, and overall lifestyle habits can influence reproductive function, hormone balance, and fertility outcomes. Adopting a balanced and nutrient-rich diet, engaging in regular physical activity, getting adequate sleep, and avoiding harmful substances can optimize reproductive health and enhance fertility potential. Additionally, alternative therapies such as acupuncture, herbal medicine, and chiropractic care can support the body's natural healing mechanisms and promote optimal functioning of the reproductive system.

3. Spirit:

The spirit encompasses the deeper dimensions of human experience, including purpose, meaning, values, and connection to something greater than oneself. For many individuals and couples, spirituality plays a significant role in their fertility journey, providing comfort, hope, and a sense of purpose amidst uncertainty and challenges. Spiritual practices such as prayer, meditation, rituals, and connection with nature can foster a sense of inner peace, resilience, and trust in the natural process of conception and birth. By nurturing the spirit, individuals can find strength, inspiration, and solace as they navigate the ups and downs of the fertility journey.

Incorporating a holistic approach that addresses mind, body, and spirit is essential for optimizing fertility outcomes and promoting overall well-being. By recognizing the interconnectedness of these elements and adopting practices that support holistic health, individuals and couples can create a fertile ground for conception, pregnancy, and the journey to parenthood. Whether through mindfulness practices, nutritional interventions, or spiritual rituals, embracing a holistic approach empowers individuals to take an active role in their fertility journey and cultivate a sense of wholeness and vitality in mind, body, and spirit.

CHAPTER 5

Navigating Emotional Challenges

A vital part of the reproductive process is navigating emotional obstacles, since individuals and couples frequently experience a rollercoaster of emotions from excitement and optimism to frustration and loss. Throughout the process, emotional resilience and well-being must be maintained by acknowledging and treating these feelings.

Stress is a typical emotional barrier to fertility that can have a detrimental effect on both the health of the reproductive system and the success of conception. Mind-body practices that assist people manage stress and foster a sense of serenity and balance include yoga, meditation, and relaxation exercises. During trying times, getting help from family, friends, support groups, or mental health specialists can also be very beneficial in terms of offering emotional support and validation.

Grief and loss are another emotional barrier to conception, especially for those who miscarry.a diagnosis of infertility, or ineffective therapy. It's crucial to give oneself permission to grieve and deal with these losses in a healthy way, whether that means keeping a journal, seeing a therapist, or taking part in rites or rituals that pay tribute to the deceased.

Relationships can be strained when navigating the ups and downs of the reproductive journey because of potential communication failures, differences in coping mechanisms, and feelings of guilt or anger. During this trying time, solid and healthy relationships must be maintained via empathy, open and honest communication, and mutual support.

In the end, overcoming emotional obstacles in fertility calls for self-compassion, endurance, and resilience. Couples and individuals can manage the fertility journey with better resilience and well-being by developing coping techniques that promote emotional well-being, getting support when necessary, and identifying and accepting their emotions.

Addressing the Emotional Rollercoaster of Fertility Struggles and Setbacks

For individuals and couples coping with infertility, addressing the emotional rollercoaster of fertility issues and setbacks is essential. There may be highs and lows on the road to conception, and it's important to recognize and accept the range of emotions that surface along the path.

1. Acknowledge and Validate emotion:

When faced with difficulties and setbacks related to fertility, it is common to feel a wide range of emotions, such as despair, frustration, anger, anxiety, and loss. The first step to effectively managing these emotions is to acknowledge and validate them. Allowing oneself to feel and express emotions in a secure and encouraging setting might encourage emotional healing and resilience as opposed to repressing or rejecting sensations.

2. Seek Support:

Asking friends, family, support groups, or mental health In trying circumstances, medical experts can offer priceless emotional support and validation. Individuals and couples might feel less alone in their journey and get perspective on their problems by having open conversations about their thoughts, sharing experiences with people who can relate, and receiving sympathetic listening.

3. Practice Self-Care:

Taking care of oneself is crucial for stress management, emotional health, and building resilience amid infertility challenges. Exercise, mindfulness, relaxation methods, hobbies, and quality time with loved ones are all beneficial for recharging, gaining perspective, and managing life's obstacles.

4. Have Reasonable Expectations:

It's critical to have reasonable expectations and accept that things could not go as to plan during the fertility process. Even though losses and disappointments might be depressing, holding onto hope and optimism can support people in overcoming adversity and remaining resilient in the face of hardship.

5. Pay Attention to What You Can control

Even though there are many aspects of the fertility journey that may seem uncontrollable, concentrating on the things that are under one's control can encourage proactive action toward one's objectives. This could entail pursuing reproductive treatments, establishing a healthy lifestyle, or supporting for oneself in medical settings, or exploring alternative paths to parenthood.

6. Practice Mindfulness and Acceptance:

Mindfulness techniques, such as meditation and mindfulness-based stress reduction, can help individuals cultivate acceptance and non-judgmental awareness of their thoughts, feelings, and bodily sensations. By staying present in the moment and practicing acceptance of the present circumstances, individuals can reduce rumination on past disappointments or anxieties about the future, leading to greater emotional resilience and well-being.

7. Seek Professional Help When Needed:

There may be times when the emotional toll of fertility struggles becomes overwhelming, and professional help from therapists, counsellors, or psychologists trained in infertility and reproductive mental health can be beneficial. These professionals can provide tailored support, coping strategies, and therapeutic interventions to help individuals and couples navigate the emotional challenges of infertility and build resilience.

8. Cultivate Hope and Resilience:

Cultivating hope and resilience is essential for weathering the ups and downs of the fertility journey. Despite setbacks and disappointments, maintaining a sense of hope, optimism, and perseverance can help individuals stay resilient and continue moving forward towards their goal of building a family, whether through biological conception, adoption, surrogacy, or other means.

In other words, addressing the emotional rollercoaster of fertility struggles and setbacks requires acknowledging and validating emotions, seeking support, practicing self-care, setting realistic expectations, focusing on what can be controlled, practicing mindfulness and acceptance, seeking professional help when needed, and cultivating hope and resilience. By implementing these strategies, individuals and couples can navigate the challenges of infertility with greater emotional well-being, strength, and resilience, ultimately empowering themselves to persevere on their journey to parenthood.

Coping Strategies and Support Systems for Women and their Partners.

The path to parenting can be exciting and full of optimism, but it can also be emotionally taxing, particularly for women and their partners who are having trouble conceiving. In order to traverse this path with resilience and wellbeing, this essay examines coping mechanisms and the several support networks that are accessible.

Strategies of Coping for Individuals

Recognize and accept your feelings: It's acceptable to experience sadness, frustration, rage, or overload. Let yourself experience your feelings without passing judgment.

- ***Take care of yourself:*** Give priority to the things that improve your physical and mental health, such working out, getting adequate sleep, eating a balanced diet, and spending time in nature.

- ***Seek out expert assistance:*** Consulting with a therapist or counselor who specializes in reproductive concerns can offer invaluable direction and assistance in handling emotions and creating coping strategies.

- ***Join a support group:*** Making connections with those going through comparable struggles can promote a feeling of shared experiences, understanding, and community.

- ***Use relaxation and mindfulness techniques:*** Stress management and emotional well-being can be enhanced by practices like yoga, meditation, and deep breathing.

- ***Keep things in perspective:*** Keep in mind that each person's experience is unique, and it can be harmful to compare your circumstances to those of others. Prioritize your own development and acknowledge little accomplishments.

Techniques for Pairs:

Honest and open communication: Let your partner know about your needs, wants, and feelings on a regular basis. Actively listen and provide assistance without passing judgment.

- ***Collective decision-making:*** Together, decide on a course of action and treatment alternatives, encouraging a sense of shared accountability and teamwork.
- ***Maintain intimacy:*** Fertility challenges can affect intimacy, but maintaining a healthy connection is crucial. Explore alternative

ways to express affection and maintain closeness.

- ***Celebrate each other:*** Acknowledge and appreciate each other's efforts and support throughout the journey.

- ***Seek couple's therapy:*** Therapy can offer valuable tools for enhancing communication, managing stress together, and strengthening your relationship.

Support Systems:

Fertility clinics and healthcare providers: These professionals can offer medical expertise, treatment options, and emotional support.

- ***Support groups:*** Online and in-person support groups connect you with others facing similar challenges, offering a sense of belonging and shared understanding.

- ***Online resources:*** There are numerous websites and online communities offering information, resources, and peer support for individuals and couples navigating fertility issues.

- ***Family and friends:*** Sharing your experiences with supportive family and friends can lessen feelings of isolation and provide a sense of belonging and understanding.

Remember:

- You are not alone. Millions of individuals and couples face fertility challenges.

- Seeking help and support is a sign of strength, not weakness.

- There is no single solution, and the best approach will vary for each individual and couple.

- Be patient with yourself and your partner, as the journey may take time.

- Focus on building resilience, maintaining emotional well-being, and navigating this challenging path together.

By implementing these coping strategies and utilizing available support systems, individuals and couples facing fertility challenges can empower themselves to navigate their journey with greater resilience, understanding, and support.

Encouraging Resilience and self-compassion throughout the Fertility Journey

Encouraging resilience and self-compassion throughout the fertility journey is essential for individuals and couples facing the challenges of infertility. Building resilience and cultivating self-compassion can help individuals navigate the emotional ups and downs of fertility struggles with greater strength, grace, and perseverance.

1. Acknowledge Strengths and Coping Skills:

Encourage individuals and couples to recognize their strengths and coping skills that have helped them navigate challenges in the past. Remind them of their resilience and ability to adapt in the face of adversity, highlighting their capacity to overcome obstacles and persevere through difficult times.

2. Practice Self-Compassion:

Encourage individuals to practice self-compassion by treating themselves with kindness, understanding, and acceptance during times of struggle. Remind them that experiencing infertility is not their fault, and it's okay to feel a range of emotions, including sadness, frustration, and grief. Encourage them to offer themselves the same compassion and support they would offer to a loved one in a similar situation.

3. Focus on Personal Growth and Healing:

Encourage individuals to view the fertility journey as an opportunity for personal growth and healing, rather than solely focusing on the outcome of conception. Encourage them to explore ways to nurture their emotional, physical, and spiritual well-being, whether through therapy, self-care practices, creative outlets, or spiritual exploration.

4. Practice Resilience-Building Strategies:

Encourage individuals to cultivate resilience by adopting coping strategies that promote emotional well-being and adaptive coping skills. This may include practicing mindfulness, seeking social support, maintaining a healthy lifestyle, setting realistic goals, reframing negative thoughts, and seeking professional help when needed.

5. Maintain Perspective and Hope:

Encourage individuals to maintain perspective and hold onto hope, even in the face of setbacks and disappointments. Remind them that infertility is just one chapter in their life story and that there are many paths to parenthood, including biological conception, adoption, surrogacy, or living a fulfilling childfree life. Encourage them to focus on the things they can control and remain open to new possibilities and opportunities.

6. Celebrate Milestones and Victories:

Encourage individuals to celebrate milestones and victories along the fertility journey, no matter how small. Whether it's completing a round of fertility treatments, reaching a personal goal, or finding moments of joy and connection amidst the challenges, encourage individuals to acknowledge and celebrate their progress and resilience along the way.

7. Offer Support and Validation:

Offer ongoing support and validation to individuals and couples as they navigate the fertility journey. Listen empathetically to their experiences, validate their emotions, and offer encouragement, understanding, and reassurance. Let them know that they are not alone and that their feelings are valid and worthy of compassion and support.

Therefore, encouraging resilience and self-compassion throughout the fertility journey is essential for helping individuals and couples navigate the emotional challenges of infertility with strength, grace, and perseverance. By acknowledging their strengths, practicing self-compassion, focusing on personal growth and healing, practicing resilience-building strategies, maintaining perspective and hope, celebrating milestones and victories, and offering support and validation, individuals and couples can cultivate resilience and self-compassion as they navigate the twists and turns of the fertility journey.

Chapter 6

Empowerment and Taking Action

Empowerment and taking action are essential principles for individuals and couples embarking on the journey of fertility. Facing challenges such as infertility or difficulty conceiving can be emotionally taxing, but by embracing empowerment and proactive engagement, individuals can navigate the complexities of fertility with resilience and determination.

Empowerment involves recognizing one's agency and ability to make informed decisions, advocate for personal needs, and actively participate in the fertility journey. Taking action goes hand in hand with empowerment, as it entails moving beyond feelings of helplessness or passivity and actively pursuing steps towards fertility goals.

In this exploration of empowerment and taking action in the context of fertility, we will delve into practical strategies, resources, and support systems that empower individuals to advocate for themselves, seek appropriate medical care, make informed decisions about treatment options, and navigate the emotional ups and downs of the fertility journey with strength and resilience. By embracing empowerment and taking proactive steps, individuals can reclaim control over their fertility journey and move forward with hope and confidence.

Encouraging women to confidently take charge of their reproductive journey is crucial to promoting resilience, autonomy, and overall wellbeing along the way. In a world where fertility issues can frequently feel overwhelming, giving women the information, tools, and support they need to make decisions, stand up for what they need, and put their physical and mental well-being first will enable them to navigate their journey with confidence.

1. Awareness and Education:

Awareness and education are the first steps toward empowerment. Giving women accurate information about reproductive health, fertility, and accessible treatments gives them the power to choose their care with knowledge. Women can take an active role in their own health by being informed about the variables that affect fertility, the different treatment options available, and the possible dangers and advantages of each to enable take an active role in their journey to fertility.

2. Access to Resources and support:

Another aspect of empowerment is making sure women have access to networks of support and resources that can assist them in overcoming the difficulties associated with infertility. This can entail having access to mental health doctors, support groups, fertility specialists, and online communities where women can interact with others who have gone through similar things. Women can find the inspiration and assurance they need to keep going when they have access to validation and support from people who have been there before.

3. Encouraging Self-Advocacy:

It is imperative to enable women to effectively advocate for their preferences and needs in medical settings. In order to make sure that their particular needs are recognized and met throughout the reproductive process, women should be encouraged to ask questions, get second opinions, and communicate their concerns and priorities to their healthcare providers. By advocating for themselves, women can ensure they receive personalized care that aligns with their values and goals.

4. Promoting Emotional Resilience:

Throughout the reproductive process, empowerment entails encouraging emotional resilience and wellbeing. Women can handle the emotional ups and downs of infertility with more resilience and strength if they are encouraged to prioritize self-care, engage in stress-reduction activities, and seek out support from family members or mental health specialists. Women who prioritize their mental well-being are more equipped to handle the obstacles they face on the journey.

5. Celebrating Agency and Choice:

At the end of the day, empowerment is about honoring women's agency and choice when it comes to becoming pregnant. Understanding that every woman's journey is different, enabling women to make decisions based on what feels right for them affirms their autonomy and self-determination, whether that decision is to pursue fertility treatments, consider other options for becoming parents, or decide not to have children. By honoring the autonomy and choices of women, we affirm their inherent worth and dignity as individuals

Finalizing with these words,enabling women to confidently take charge of their reproductive journeys entails giving them the knowledge, tools, support, and encouragement they need to prioritize their well-being, speak up for themselves, make educated decisions, and celebrate their agency and choices. By giving women the confidence to take charge of their fertility journey, we celebrate their tenacity, fortitude, and ability to carve out fulfilling paths to parenting on their own terms.

Providing Practical Steps and Action Plans for Pursuing Fertility Goals

Providing practical steps and action plans for pursuing fertility goals is essential in helping individuals and couples navigate the complex journey of fertility with clarity, confidence, and purpose. By breaking down the process into manageable steps and offering concrete strategies for taking action, individuals can feel empowered to move forward towards their fertility goals with greater agency and determination. Here are some practical steps and action plans for pursuing fertility goals:

1. Consultation with Fertility Specialist:

Schedule an initial consultation with a fertility specialist to discuss your fertility goals, medical history, and any concerns or questions you may have. This appointment will provide valuable information about your reproductive health and help you understand your options for achieving pregnancy.

2. Fertility Testing:

Undergo comprehensive fertility testing to assess your reproductive health and identify any potential barriers to conception. This may include blood tests to evaluate hormone levels, imaging studies to assess ovarian reserve and uterine health, and semen analysis for male partners.

3. Lifestyle Modifications:

Make lifestyle modifications to optimize your fertility potential. This may include maintaining a healthy weight, adopting a balanced diet rich in nutrients, getting regular exercise, avoiding tobacco, alcohol, and recreational drugs, managing stress, and getting adequate sleep.

4. *Exploring Treatment Options:*

Explore various treatment options available to help you achieve pregnancy. Depending on your individual circumstances, this may include timed intercourse, intrauterine insemination (IUI), in vitro fertilization (IVF), or other assisted reproductive technologies (ART).

5. *Financial Planning:*

Develop a financial plan to cover the costs associated with fertility testing and treatment. Research insurance coverage, savings accounts, payment plans, and financing options to determine the most feasible approach for financing your fertility journey.

6. *Emotional Support:*

Seek emotional support from loved ones, support groups, or mental health professionals to cope with the emotional challenges of fertility struggles. Connecting with others who understand your experiences can provide validation, encouragement, and a sense of community.

7. *Self-Care Practices:*

Prioritize self-care practices to support your emotional and physical well-being during the fertility journey. This may include mindfulness meditation, relaxation techniques, journaling, engaging in hobbies or creative outlets, and taking breaks when needed.

8. *Follow-Up Appointments:*

Schedule follow-up appointments with your fertility specialist to review test results, discuss treatment options, and make any necessary adjustments to your fertility plan. Regular communication with your healthcare team will ensure that you stay informed and supported throughout your fertility journey.

9. Consider Alternative Paths to Parenthood:

Explore alternative paths to parenthood, such as adoption, surrogacy, or donor options, if conventional fertility treatments are not successful or feasible for you. Keep an open mind and consider all available options for building your family.

10.Maintain Hope and Resilience:

Lastly, maintain hope and resilience throughout your fertility journey, even in the face of setbacks and challenges. Remember that every individual's journey is unique, and there are many paths to parenthood. Stay focused on your goals, lean on your support network, and believe in your ability to overcome obstacles and achieve your dreams of starting or expanding your family.

By following these practical steps and action plans, individuals and couples can navigate the complexities of the fertility journey with confidence, clarity, and purpose. Each step brings them closer to their fertility goals and empowers them to take control of their reproductive health and well-being.

Encouraging proactive communication with healthcare providers and fertility specialists

Encouraging proactive communication with healthcare providers and fertility specialists is crucial for individuals and couples navigating the fertility journey. Open and effective communication fosters trust, collaboration, and personalized care, ultimately leading to better outcomes and experiences. Here are some key reasons why proactive communication with healthcare providers is important:

- ***Sharing Concerns and Preferences:*** Proactive communication allows individuals and couples to share their concerns, preferences, and priorities with their healthcare providers. Whether it's discussing treatment options, expressing emotional or logistical challenges, or voicing cultural or religious considerations, open communication ensures that healthcare decisions align with the individual's values and goals.

- ***Understanding Treatment Options:*** Effective communication ensures that individuals and couples have a clear understanding of their treatment options, including the potential risks, benefits, success rates, and alternatives. By discussing the pros and cons of each option, healthcare providers can help individuals make informed decisions that are tailored to their unique needs and circumstances.

- ***Clarifying Expectations and Goals:*** Proactive communication allows individuals and couples to clarify their expectations and goals for fertility treatment. Whether it's discussing the likelihood of success, the anticipated timeline, or the potential financial costs involved, open dialogue ensures that everyone is on the same page and working towards a shared understanding of the desired outcomes.

- ***Monitoring Progress and Adjusting Plans:*** Regular communication with healthcare providers allows for ongoing monitoring of progress and adjustment of treatment plans as needed. By staying in touch with their providers and reporting any changes or concerns, individuals can ensure that their care remains responsive to their evolving needs and circumstances.

- ***Maximizing Understanding and Collaboration:*** Proactive communication ensures that individuals and couples fully understand their fertility diagnosis, treatment options, and care plan. Encourage them to ask questions, seek clarification, and actively participate in discussions with their healthcare providers. This collaborative approach fosters a deeper understanding of the fertility journey and empowers individuals to make informed decisions about their care.

- ***Building Trust and Rapport:*** Open communication builds trust and rapport between patients and healthcare providers.

Encourage individuals to share their concerns, preferences, and expectations openly with their providers. By establishing a supportive and trusting relationship, individuals can feel more comfortable discussing sensitive topics and expressing their needs throughout the fertility process.

- ***Addressing Emotional and Psychological Needs:*** Proactive communication allows individuals to address their emotional and psychological needs during the fertility journey. Encourage them to communicate any fears, anxieties, or emotional challenges they may be experiencing with their healthcare team. This open dialogue enables providers to offer appropriate support, resources, and referrals to mental health professionals if needed.

- ***Optimizing Treatment Outcomes:*** Effective communication with healthcare providers can optimize treatment outcomes. Encourage individuals to report any changes or concerns regarding their symptoms, side effects, or response to treatment promptly. This allows providers to make timely adjustments to the treatment plan and ensure that individuals receive the best possible care for their unique needs.

- ***Advocating for Personalized Care:*** Proactive communication empowers individuals to advocate for personalized care that aligns with their values, preferences, and lifestyle. Encourage them to voice their treatment goals, priorities, and any cultural or religious considerations that may impact their care. By actively participating in their care decisions, individuals can ensure that their treatment plan is tailored to meet their individual needs and circumstances.

- ***Education and Support:*** Encourage individuals to stay informed about their fertility journey by seeking reliable information from trusted sources and attending educational events or support groups. Proactive communication with healthcare providers also provides opportunities for ongoing education and support throughout the fertility process.

In summary, proactive communication with healthcare providers and fertility specialists is essential for maximizing understanding, building trust, addressing emotional needs, optimizing treatment outcomes, advocating for personalized care, and continuing education and support throughout the fertility journey. Encouraging individuals and couples to actively engage with their healthcare team empowers them to take control of their fertility care and achieve the best possible outcome.

Chapter 7

Real Stories of Triumph

Real Stories of Triumph offers a touching exploration of the human experience within the realm of fertility struggles. In this collection, we delve into the lived experiences of individuals and couples who have faced the challenges of infertility with courage, resilience, and hope. Through their stories, we gain insight into the emotional rollercoaster of fertility struggles, the complexities of medical interventions, and the profound impact of perseverance and resilience on the journey to parenthood.

Each story is a testament to the strength of the human spirit and the power of resilience in the face of adversity. From the initial heartache of receiving a diagnosis to the triumph of holding a long-awaited baby in their arms, these narratives offer a glimpse into the highs and lows, the joys and sorrows, and the moments of grace and resilience that characterize the fertility journey.

Through the lens of personal narratives, "Real Stories of Triumph" aims to inspire, educate, and uplift readers who may be navigating their own fertility journey or supporting a loved one through similar challenges. By sharing these stories of triumph, we seek to foster understanding, empathy, and connection within the broader community, while also celebrating the resilience and strength of those who have walked the path of infertility and emerged victorious.

In the pages that follow, you will encounter stories of hope, resilience, and ultimately, triumph in the face of adversity. These stories remind us that while the journey to parenthood may be fraught with challenges, it is also filled with moments of beauty, grace, and profound transformation. May these real stories of triumph serve as beacons of hope and inspiration for all who embark on the journey of fertility.

Babies after 40: Three moms' stories

Recently I attended a delivery of a baby a baby born to a mother who was almost 50 years old. I did a double-take when I saw her age on the chart– this was the oldest mother I had ever seen deliver. Her baby, who had Down Syndrome, seemed like a miracle to her.

These are the stories of three other women who conceived babies after age 40– three other women ecstatic to conceive so late in life.

A woman's chances of conception start to fall around age 25, and by age 45 healthy women without known infertility have only about a 5% chance of becoming pregnant. The risks associated with late-in-life pregnancy are significant for both mother and child. Yet the women I spoke with all seemed very willing to accept these risks. Here are their stories of loss, sacrifice, and joy.

Lilli, conceived at age 46

With a history of six miscarriages including three after age 40, Lilli and her husband were no strangers to loss. She delivered her last miscarried baby at home, a perfectly formed tiny human she was able to see, hold, and grieve for with her husband and four living children. They named him and had a private family funeral. The likelihood of another child seemed bleak. And so they opened their home to two foster children – brothers, one with special needs.

And then those foster children also left their home, leaving another sense of emptiness, another hurt, another loss. Just days later, Lilli was conceived, naturally, without the aid of infertility treatments. She was 46. This was an unexpected joy. Her whole family was starting to heal.

There was no shortage of medical concerns. Lilli had to address her gluten sensitivity and make big changes to her diet. She had to get healthy quickly. And it worked– she had a healthy pregnancy, healthy natural delivery, and healthy baby, all at the age of 46.

Her oldest child was already 14 years old, busy taking selfies and acting like a self-centered teenager. When the baby came, the selfies turned to selflessness. "Love never divides," Lilli said, "It only multiplies."

Nancy, conceived at age 41

Nancy's friends didn't really believe that she had infertility, she had four healthy children. Yet she hadn't conceived in nearly 7 years despite a happy marriage and the absence of birth control. And then, at 39, she naturally conceived her fifth child. And again, to her delight, she conceived her sixth child at age 41, also without the aid of infertility treatment.

Nancy's husband, Mark, was 46 when they conceived their 6th child. Nancy started to calculate his age when the baby graduated from high school. "Let's not even do the math," Mark said.

"Every time I went to the doctor it seemed like they were trying to scare me," she said. Although Nancy appreciated her doctor's care and concern, it just seemed like no one understood her delight and the obvious reasons why she was willing to accept all these medical risks. Other than some high blood pressure, her pregnancy and delivery were healthy. So is her baby.

Nancy is now a mother of six children ages 19, 17, 12, 10, 3 and 1. What's different now compared to when she was a 20-something-mom? "I'm tired more," she said, but she has lots of help from her older children, who adore the baby.

People have started mistaking Nancy as the grandmother of her infant, especially when she goes out shopping with her 19-year-old daughter and the baby. When she clarified her status as mother, one cashier remarked, "That's dangerous." Nancy wonders if people would be so critical if this were her first child.

Mary, conceived at age 44 (delivered at 45)

"I nearly died with my 4th baby due to high blood pressure. I saw a specialist, one of the best doctors in Boston, and he told me never to get pregnant again, because if I did it could be fatal to both me and the baby." Then, she found out she was pregnant at age 45. "My doctor told me I was the oldest patient in his practice." Yet he supported Mary 100%, never criticizing her for choosing to carry her baby. He warned Mary to anticipate months of bedrest, but fortunately she had only one week of bedrest before she delivered a very healthy baby boy after an easy labor and delivery.

"The amazing thing was that I was really healthy through my 5th pregnancy. I had more problems with my other pregnancies when I was younger."

Mary is now 54 with an 8 year old. "I'm much more relaxed now, as a mom." She says she doesn't feel very old– she has to think about her age, even though her oldest is 24 and she is a grandmother. "A lot of women my age are all done with children. Having children keeps me young and active. I'm less focused on myself, less selfish."

The world is full of criticism of people's parenting choices. I've been widely criticized for having five children. Behind every hard decision is a story.

Diverse Paths to Parenthood and the Resilience of the Human Spirit

The book "Real Stories of Triumph" honors the variety of routes to parenting as well as the human spirit's extraordinary fortitude in the face of infertility difficulties. Readers are invited to observe the fortitude, bravery, and tenacity of individuals and couples as they traverse the challenges of infertility through a tapestry of personal accounts.

These tales highlight the variety of ways that people start families, from traditional methods like IVF and surrogacy to non-traditional routes like adoption and donor choices. Every story is an ode to the steadfast wish to become a parent and the inventive ways people find to realize their aspirations of beginning or growing a family.

These tales also highlight how resilient the human spirit can be, even in the face of hardships and disappointments. In spite of These individuals and couples exhibit an amazing ability to survive, adapt, and find optimism even in the most difficult circumstances, in spite of encountering unfathomable hurdles. Their tales encourage us to trust in the tenacity of people, serving as a constant reminder that despite hardship, people can rise above it.

"Real Stories of Triumph" honors variety, resiliency, and the strength of the human spirit that never fades. Readers are invited to witness the tenacious spirit that is within each of us, the transformational journey of parenthood, and the beauty of the human experience through these stories.

Providing Hope and Encouragement to Readers facing Similar Challenges

For readers going through comparable difficulties with conception, "Real Stories of Triumph" is a source of inspiration and hope. Readers are reminded that they are not alone in their challenges and that there is hope through the genuine and unvarnished stories presented within its pages.

Every narrative provides a ray of hope by highlighting the fortitude, bravery, and tenacity of people and couples who have braved the trials of infertility and come out stronger on the other side. These accounts, which range from the first heartbreaking diagnosis to the ultimate happiness of holding a newborn in their arms, demonstrate that miracles may occur even in the face of uncertainty and hopelessness.

Through openness and sensitivity in discussing their experiences, they are actively pursuing reproductive treatments, investigating alternate routes to parenthood, or simply finding solace in the experiences of others.

More than just a compilation of tales, "Real Stories of Triumph" is a monument to the ability of the human spirit to triumph against misfortune. It is a source of hope, encouragement, and inspiration for all who dare to dream of building a family against all odds.

Conclusion

As we reach the conclusion of ",The Fertility Solution: Fertility Secrets for the Modern Woman Over 40" it's important to reflect on the key insights, strategies, and empowering fertility secrets that have been shared throughout the book. From the courageous narratives of individuals and couples facing infertility to the empowering strategies for navigating the fertility journey, each chapter has offered valuable wisdom and inspiration for readers.

Throughout the book, we have learned that the fertility journey is as unique as the individuals who embark upon it. There is no one-size-fits-all approach, and each person's path to parenthood may be different. However, there are common themes that emerge – resilience, hope, and the unwavering belief in the possibility of miracles.

We have explored diverse paths to parenthood, from conventional fertility treatments to alternative options such as adoption and surrogacy. We have witnessed the power of proactive communication with healthcare providers, the importance of self-care and emotional support, and the transformative impact of embracing one's fertility journey with courage and optimism.

As we conclude our journey together, I encourage you, dear reader, to embrace your fertility journey with courage and optimism. Know that you are not alone – there is a community of individuals and couples who understand your struggles and are rooting for your success. Lean on your loved ones for support, seek guidance from trusted healthcare providers, and never lose sight of the hope that lies within you.

Remember, the fertility journey is not just about achieving a positive pregnancy test – it's about embracing the journey itself, with all its twists and turns, joys and sorrows. It's about finding meaning and purpose in the challenges we face and emerging stronger and more resilient on the other side.

As you move forward on your fertility journey, hold onto hope, persevere in the face of adversity, and believe in your fertility potential. Miracles do happen, and your dreams of parenthood are within reach. May you find the strength, courage, and belief in yourself to navigate this journey with grace and resilience.

In closing, let us celebrate the transformative power of hope, perseverance, and belief in our fertility potential. May each of us find the courage to embrace our fertility journey with optimism and faith, knowing that our triumphs are just around the corner.

Recommended Resources

General Fertility:

- ***The Infertility Handbook:*** How to Understand and Manage Your Fertility Problems by Diane M. Barnes and Lynn M. Westphal

- ***It Starts with the Egg:*** How the Science of Eggs Can Help You Get Pregnant Naturally by Rebecca Fett

- ***The Complete Guide to Getting Pregnant:*** Understanding Your Body and Maximizing Your Chances of Conception by Natalie Berger

- ***The Baby Decision:*** How to Make the Most Important Decision of Your Life by Merle Bombardieri

- ***Fertility After 40:*** What to Expect When You're Expecting After 40 by Heidi Murkoff and Sharon Mazel

- ***Conceiving at the Crossroads:*** Your Guide to Fertility After 35 by Alice D. Domar

- ***The New Our Bodies, Ourselves:*** A Revolutionary Guide to Women's Health by Boston Women's Health Book Collective

The Essential Guide to Getting Pregnant After 35 by Zita West

Mind-Body Connection:

- ***Mind Body Baby:*** Conception, Pregnancy and Birth by Carole Myles

- ***The Fertile Mind:*** How to Manage Stress and Optimize Your Reproductive Health for a Healthy Pregnancy by Dr. Alice Domar

- ***The Power of Your Mind:*** How to Use the Power of Your Mind to Change Your Life by Louise Hay

Web Resources:

- Resolve: The National Infertility Association: https://resolve.org/
- The American Society for Reproductive Medicine (ASRM): https://www.asrm.org/
- The National Council on Family Relations (NCFR): https://www.ncfr.org/
- Fertility Network: https://fertilitynetworkuk.org/ (UK-based, but offers valuable resources)
- The National Center for Complementary and Integrative Health (NCCIH): https://www.nccih.nih.gov/health (Offers information on various holistic practices)